THE
DIABETES
AIR FRYER
COOKBOOK

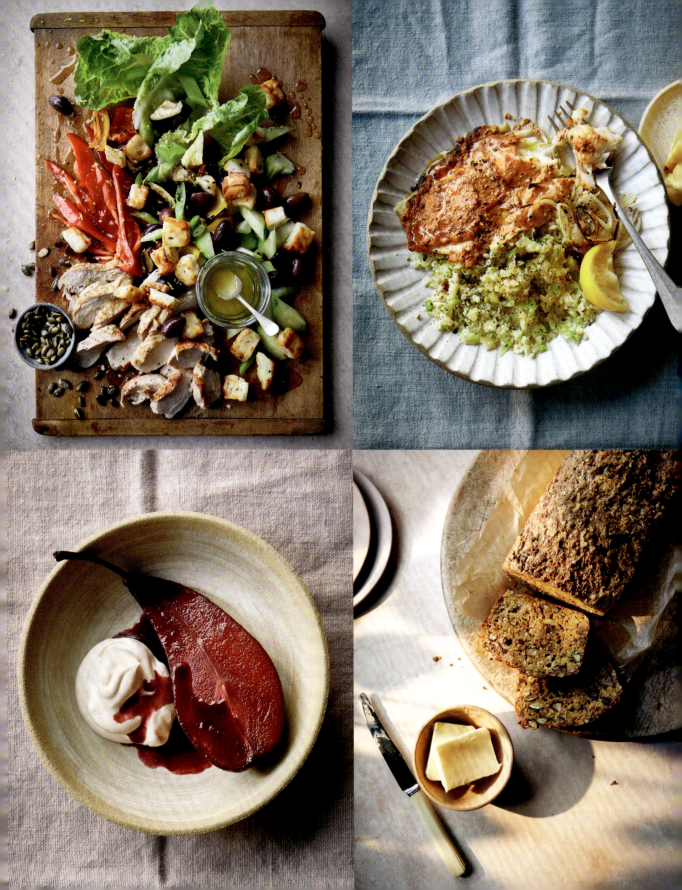

THE DIABETES AIR FRYER COOKBOOK

EASY, EVERYDAY RECIPES TO LOSE WEIGHT AND BEAT TYPE 2 DIABETES

KATIE CALDESI

With Dr David Unwin, Dr Jen Unwin and Jenny Phillips

hamlyn

First published in Great Britain in 2025 by Hamlyn,
an imprint of Octopus Publishing Group Ltd
Carmelite House
50 Victoria Embankment
London EC4Y 0DZ
www.octopusbooks.co.uk
www.octopusbooksusa.com

An Hachette UK Company
www.hachette.co.uk

The authorized representative in the EEA is Hachette
Ireland, 8 Castlecourt Centre, Castleknock Road,
Castleknock, Dublin 15, D15 YF6A, Ireland
(email: info@hbgi.ie)

Distributed in the US by Hachette Book Group
1290 Avenue of the Americas, 4th and 5th Floors
New York, NY 10104

Distributed in Canada by Canadian Manda Group
664 Annette St., Toronto, Ontario, Canada M6S 2C8

ISBN 978-0-600-63896-4

A CIP catalogue record for this book is available from
the British Library.

Printed and bound in China.

10 9 8 7 6 5 4 3 2 1

Publisher: Kate Fox
Editor: Scarlet Furness
Copy Editor: Claire Rogers
Art Director: Yasia Williams
Designer: Paul Palmer-Edwards
Photographer: Maja Smend
Food Stylist: Lizzie Harris
Prop Stylist: Tony Hutchinson
Assistant Production Manager: Lisa Pinnell

Standard level spoon measurements are used in all recipes.

1 tablespoon = one 15ml spoon

1 teaspoon = one 5ml spoon

The Department of Health advises that eggs should not be consumed raw. This book contains dishes made with raw or lightly cooked eggs. It is prudent for more vulnerable people such as pregnant and nursing mothers, the elderly, babies and young children to avoid uncooked or lightly cooked dishes made with eggs. Once prepared, these dishes should be kept refrigerated and used promptly.

Milk should be full fat unless otherwise stated.

Fresh herbs should be used unless otherwise stated. If unavailable, use dried herbs as an alternative but halve the quantities stated.

Pepper should be freshly ground black pepper unless otherwise stated.

This book includes dishes made with nuts and nut derivatives. It is advisable for those with known allergic reactions to nuts and nut derivatives and those who may be potentially vulnerable to these allergies, such as pregnant and nursing mothers, the elderly, babies and children, to avoid dishes made with nuts and nut oils.

It is also prudent to check the labels of pre-prepared ingredients for the possible inclusion of nut derivatives.

Vegetarians should look for the 'V' symbol on a cheese to ensure it is made with vegetarian rennet.

Nutritional analysis is only a guide. Brands vary, software has glitches, such as when fat is drained away but still calculated, bones are sometimes in or out of a weight.

Key to icons

 Contains Fish

 Contains Meat

 Vegetarian

 Freezes Well

 Budget Friendly

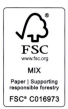

Contents

Introduction

Sceptic to Air Fryer Girl: Katie's journey into air frying

'There is so much you can do in an air fryer,' 23-year-old student Charlotte told me when I first ordered one. I was yet to be convinced that I needed another gadget that I had coped without for years as a cookery writer. It would have to compete with work surface real estate along with my food processor and toaster, but after just a couple of days, I was hooked. Their speed, the energy saved and the easy clean-up are just a few of the things I love about them; I've gone from complete sceptic to being called 'air-fryer girl' by my friends.

Charlotte loves her air fryer for quick, inexpensive meals. She is vegetarian so chose an air fryer with two drawers, one for her veggie meals and the other for cooking meat for her boyfriend. Other air fryer enthusiasts I know include a friend living alone, who chose a small, single-drawer option; and a couple who have become empty nesters yet whose kids come home at the weekend – they chose one with a removable drawer for maximum capacity. Unless you are always cooking for more than four people, air fryers have a place in everyone's kitchen, and they are here to stay. In the UK alone, more than 50 per cent of households own an air fryer.

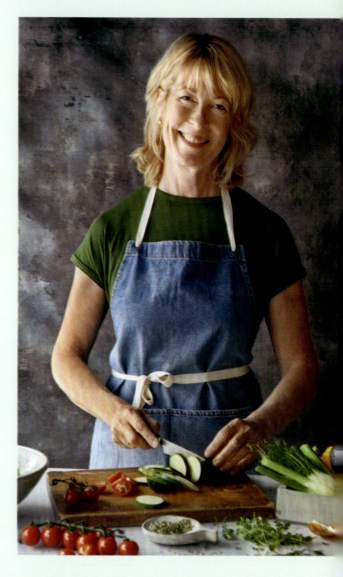

Going beyond the beige!

I used to think that using an air fryer wasn't for me, as I am always telling people to avoid eating beige, fried food; but there I was, looking at a gadget that fries... or so I thought. Fried foods are often full of sugar, starch and poor-quality fats, so I was worried. However, I now know that air fryers can cook a huge array of wonderfully colourful meals in minutes, as well as healthy versions of classics such as fried chicken and chips.

My mantra when writing this book was that if a recipe was not made healthier, faster or more convenient by cooking it in an air fryer, then it wouldn't be included. With convoluted means, it is possible to cook almost anything in an air fryer, but that shouldn't be the point. When you need large quantities or top and bottom heat together, the conventional oven wins. When you need to constantly watch what you are cooking or you want water or wine to evaporate, the hob wins. However, an air fryer wins on speed, cost, energy usage, washing up and making things crispy and crunchy. Therefore, I have concentrated on recipes that are particularly well-suited to being cooked in an air fryer and that make easy, tasty foods that should provide minimal glucose spikes.

How can an air fryer help control type 2 diabetes?

If air fryers get you cooking simple meals from scratch that are lower in carbohydrates rather than ordering fried foods from a delivery app or buying ultra-processed foods, they can help you to become healthier, slimmer and more energetic.

My husband, Giancarlo, is in his twelfth year of remission from type 2 diabetes; all of his success has been from his change in food choices; he has never been on medication. He is an Italian chef and restaurateur who loved his pasta, sugary cappuccinos and pastries a little too much and his health suffered greatly. Now he follows a low-carb lifestyle. He has kept off 4 stone (56 pounds) of weight; he has got rid of his arthritis, gout, constant hunger and exhaustion; and his eyesight and mobility have improved. In fact, he runs around like an energetic young man and yet he is 73 years old. If he can do it, anyone can.

Our principle is to cook low-carb meals, which broadly follows the pre-1950s Mediterranean diet: plenty of fresh seasonal vegetables, extra-virgin olive oil, meat, fish, eggs and dairy. Air fryers came out when low-fat cooking was still fashionable, whereas I often preserve good fats to enrich flavour and provide satiety. We aren't fatphobic! With type 2 diabetes in mind, these recipes are all about avoiding sugar and swapping out starchy foods that easily break down into sugar for wholesome, healthy alternatives to help lessen blood sugar spikes – and that will help keep diabetes under control.

Getting confident

Air fryers make cooking simple; you just need to choose a temperature and time, and you're off! If you are new to them, start by cooking a piece of bacon and a tomato or salmon with some roasted Mediterranean vegetables. You will be making meals in no time. At first you can check the food regularly, so you avoid any mistakes.

No waste

By cooking single or two portions of food you are less likely to make more than you need. Air fryers are great for cooking food from frozen, which means you can simply pull out one fish fillet or piece of chicken at a time. Do make swaps for something you already have in the refrigerator. Because I cook small amounts of food in an air fryer, I don't have so many leftovers, so there are no second helpings to be tempted by. If you do happen to have any leftovers, save them in containers in the refrigerator and use the handy 'reheat' setting to warm them thoroughly.

Budget recipes

These recipes are a great way to make delicious, healthy food on a budget. There are so many ways to save money when cooking, including buying own brands from supermarkets, using frozen options for meat, fish, vegetables and berries, shopping at markets in season and buying in bulk. It's also a good idea to freeze leftover seeds and nuts to stop them going rancid.

Other tips are to keep a pot of rosemary and thyme on a windowsill outdoors to use regularly rather than buying packets each time, freezing leftover cheeses such as mozzarella and feta from a block for re-use, and in recipes such as Roasted Mediterranean Vegetables (see page 138), use more of inexpensive vegetables which are in season and omit more expensive ones.

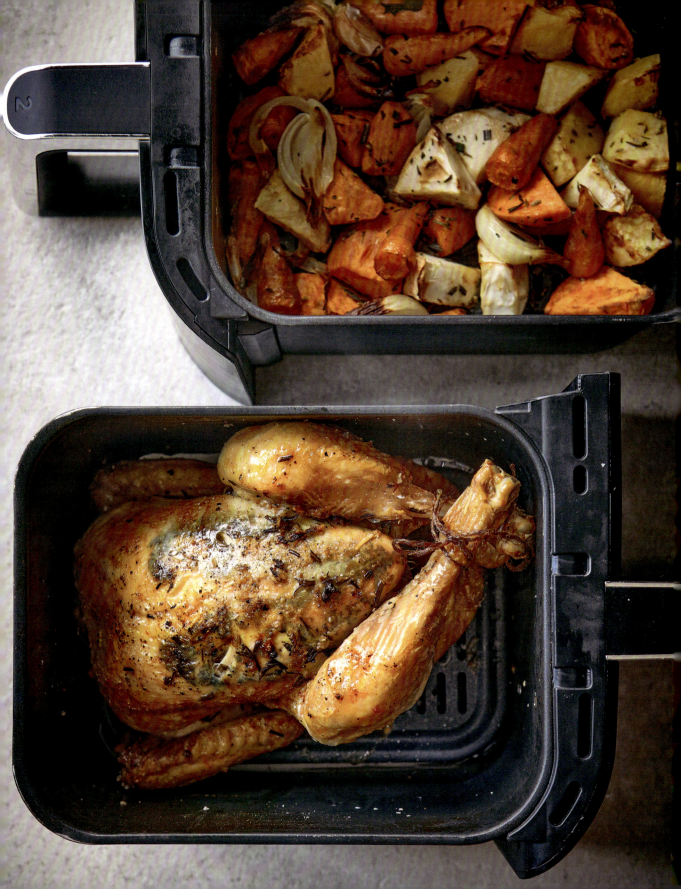

How To Use Your Air Fryer

What is an air fryer and which type should you choose?

An air fryer is a mini oven with a powerful fan allowing food to be cooked at up to twice the usual speed of a convection oven. As they were used as a low-fat way to cook chips instead of deep-fat frying them, they became known as 'air fryers', but really they can cook anything that is usually baked, roasted, grilled, steamed or fried.

The heat comes from an element at the top and is forced around the chamber by a powerful fan. Imagine a hot whirlwind under the scorching sun and you'll get the idea. Food crispens from all around provided the air can circulate freely. Most air fryers have one or two drawers. Some air fryers are more like mini ovens with trays on shelves, and there are halogen air fryers that rotate a plate of food (these are generally slower).

Go big! Even if you are only cooking for one on most days, a small air fryer with a single drawer can cause frustration. I like the dual drawer ones, so I can cook my veg separately to my meat. If space is an issue, choose one that has one drawer on top of another rather than side by side, so they take up less of that precious counter space. If you are cooking for a family, go for one with a large capacity. Some air fryers do synchronized cooking, so two batches can be cooked at the same time and some have a divider that can be removed for big roasts.

How fast are they really, and do they save energy?

Air fryers are fast. Trust me. I didn't appreciate how fast they could be and did my usual thing of putting something into cook while I brushed my teeth or answered the phone, only to return and find I had burned whatever I had been cooking.

Until you are confident of your timings, err on the side of caution and check the food regularly.

Air fryers often cook 20 per cent quicker than conventional ovens. Their smaller spaces are faster to heat up. This means that along with quick cook or no-preheat capabilities, air fryers can save one-third of the energy used by conventional ovens. And I am being cautious with these numbers; many manufacturers claim to save you up to 65 per cent.

They often save meal prep time too, as frozen food often doesn't need defrosting before being cooked in an air fryer. Sausages, for example, can be cooked in around 15 minutes from frozen.

Cooking times

It should be noted that my suggested cooking times are only a guide. The time will vary depending on the size of the ingredients; for example, a large chicken breast will take longer to cook than a small one, and it takes longer for heat to penetrate through a thicker piece of fish than a flatter tail fillet.

Air fryers differ too. My cooking times have been tested in two different air fryers, but both are fast, around 2470W, and have a capacity of around 9 litres (16 pints). If your air fryer is slower, you may need to add up to 3 minutes to my cooking times. You will soon work it out if you cook something straightforward, like a rasher of bacon or a piece of salmon.

These recipes were tested in a Ninja Foodi MAX Dual Zone 9.5L air fryer and a Salter 9L Dual Air Fryer, XL Capacity air fryer. Both have two drawers and crisper plates. Timings may vary for other brands. If you have an air fryer with a paddle,

I suggest removing it for ease of following the instructions in these recipes.

Different settings and fan speeds

Most air fryers have the capacity to lower the fan speed; settings such as 'max crisp' or 'air fry' tend to be higher than 'reheat' or 'rehydrate'. It's not always obvious or stated in the instructions, so listen to your air fryer and you will hear the speed and strength of the fan slow for certain settings. I have referenced this in the Hot Chocolate Soufflé on page 179.

Tips and tricks for air-fryer cooking

· Although wet foods need to be contained in a liner, the more you use the crisper, the better the results, as the air can get to the base of the food. They aren't hard to wash, and most can go into a dishwasher, so don't always go for a lazy disposable liner!

· To speed up cooking further, use a rack to raise the food up so it is nearer the heat.

· To fry in oil or cook anything 'wet', you will need an ovenproof dish or silicone liner without holes, or you can simply use the base of the drawer if it is flat.

· Shake, toss or turn the ingredients halfway through cooking.

· When you are spraying oil inside, tilt the drawer so that the oil bottle is always vertical; this means the spray bottle will work better.

What you *can't* do in an air fryer – and what to be careful of

You can't successfully boil food or cook large quantities of wet foods like a casserole, as the liquid can't evaporate enough, so they can't reduce to concentrate the flavour.

You can't cook food with a very wet batter, such as fish, as it drips through the holes in the racks. Therefore, breadcrumbed food is better than battered in an air fryer.

You can cook cakes, but they need to be protected with tin foil wrapped securely around them, so the outside doesn't burn before the inside is done.

Watch out! A hot oven cooks quicker than one heating up from cold. And so will a hot air fryer cook more quickly than a cold one. If you have just been cooking in it – for instance when batch cooking – foods might cook up to a couple of minutes quicker (due to the retained heat).

Don't let food fly around! Don't let food get too close to the heating element or it could be a fire risk. So, no loose herbs or flaked almonds, and no loose paper or tin foil. You also have to beware of baking paper, light food such as crispy kale leaves and grated or thinly sliced cheese flying up into the heating element. A rack can be used to hold food down.

A crowded space may take longer. One very small chicken will cook in around 35 minutes but two may take up to 45 minutes, as the heat doesn't circulate around as efficiently. Don't overfill the air fryer, the air needs to circulate evenly around the food, so a single layer of food is best.

Make sure your air fryer has plenty of space around it so the fan works well. Don't use it in a cupboard or under a work surface.

Do you need to pre heat?

Usually this is unnecessary as these small, powerful ovens heat up very quickly, though I have mentioned to pre heat in some recipes when it is essential the food goes into a hot space. If your air fryer is not powerful, then heat the empty air fryer for 4 minutes before putting the food inside. Some ovens will beep when they are ready to cook.

How to clean your air fryer

Cooking smells and fat splashes around the hob are a thing of the past, but do treat your air fryer with love! Don't let anyone touch your air fryer with a metal utensil. The non-stick coating that is so easy to clean will start to rub off. Wash it after each time you use it. Otherwise, old cooking juices left at the bottom may burn the next time you use it. Most parts, including the drawers, can be washed in a dishwasher, but do check the manufacturer's instructions.

Cooking meat safely in an air fryer

Since most cooking instructions in non-air fryer cookbooks don't mention air fryer cooking times (yet!), I recommend buying an instant-read temperature probe to test the internal temperature of cooked food. Although models of air fryers differ, generally they cook more quickly than conventional ovens. You don't want to overcook and dry meat and fish, so use this easy guide to check if your food is done.

A digital temperature probe is inexpensive and is simple to use. Simply push the tip of the probe into the thickest piece or area of meat or fish and read the temperature on the screen. The UK Food Standards Agency suggests that cooked meat should show a temperature of 75°C (167°F) for at least 30 seconds. The Food and Drug Administration (FDA) in the US suggests it reaches 74°C (165°F).

If you don't have a thermometer, simply cut the biggest piece or thickest area of meat and check that the juices run clear. In chicken, there should also be no sign of pink flesh or pink juices.

With pieces of meat such as steaks, cutlets and roasting joints (not rolled joints), usually only the surface can be contaminated. Make sure the surface is properly cooked and sealed to kill any bacteria, even if the middle of the meat is still pink. See the recipes for further details on how to tell when the meat is done.

Cooking fish safely in an air fryer

The thickness of fish is important when cooking in an air fryer. A tail piece that is only a couple of centimetres (less than an inch) thick will cook through more quickly than a piece of cod measuring 4cm (1½ inches), so the cooking times are a guide rather than a strict rule. To check if the fish is cooked, official UK and US food regulation websites, such as the FDA, state it should be opaque all the way through (no longer translucent), be firm to the touch, not wobbly and flakes should separate easily with a fork.

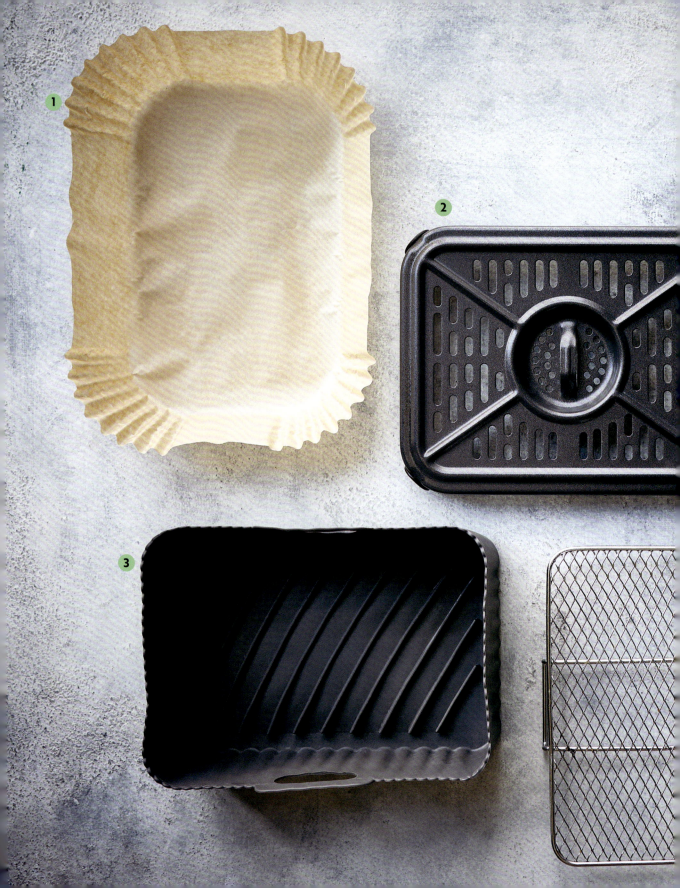

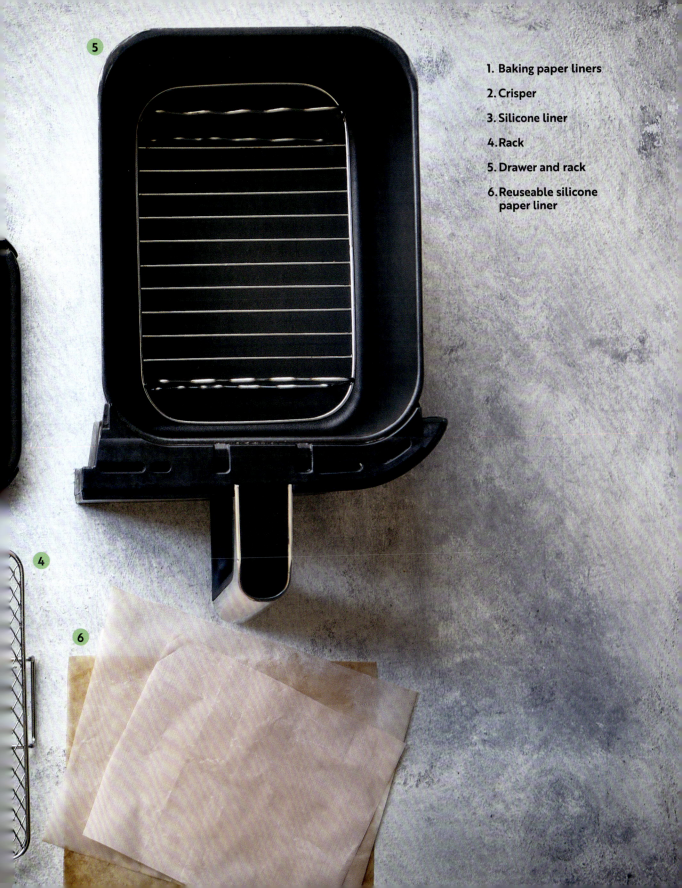

1. **Baking paper liners**

2. **Crisper**

3. **Silicone liner**

4. **Rack**

5. **Drawer and rack**

6. **Reuseable silicone paper liner**

Air Fryer Staples and Equipment

My staple ingredients – what's in my kitchen cupboard and refrigerator

Eggs: I use mixed sizes, so I don't specify the size unless it really matters to a recipe if your egg is small or very large.

Extra-virgin olive oil

Butter: salted or unsalted

Fine or flaked sea salt and freshly ground black pepper

Fresh or frozen garlic

Spring onions: great for cooking in small quantities

Vanilla extract

Ground almonds: buy in big bags or grind your own

Fresh chillies or dried chilli flakes or powder: I can't be prescriptive about the amount needed for each recipe, as the heat of chillies differs so much; you have to taste them and add accordingly. Remember, the heat is in the pith, not the seeds.

What oil or fat to use

Choose the traditional fat used in the country of the recipe's origin. For example, don't try cooking an Italian Bolognese with coconut oil, but do use coconut oil for a great base flavour if you are making a Thai curry. Extra-virgin olive oil, butter, tallow (beef fat), coconut oil and avocado oil are our favourite fats for cooking. To save money, use a refillable spray bottle for the olive or avocado oil and save chicken, bacon or meat fat from a roast to re-use, just like our grandmothers did – it's delicious and already paid for.

Sweeteners

Jenny, Jen and David would tell you to give desserts a miss on a low-carb lifestyle, especially when you are trying to curb your sugar cravings and lose weight. However, if you feel you can cope with the occasional treat, as Giancarlo does, there are some decadent desserts for special occasions and petite puddings that are low carb and still taste amazing.

Overall, I have reduced the sweetness in the dessert recipes. This is because, like many people, I have become 'low sugar adapted', as we have tried to eliminate sugar from our diets. Over time, even for sugar addicts like my husband, Giancarlo, our sweet tooth changes and a shop-bought cake that was once pleasant becomes sickly sweet.

Even if you use dates or honey, the amounts I use in these recipes are still so much lower than in commercially-made puddings, so you will be reducing your carb intake by making dessert at home. I give the option to use minimal dates, honey or erythritol, a sugar alcohol sweetener that has zero net carbs in terms of sugar and zero calories.

Allulose is expensive and although it has been approved by the FDA in America, it is still going through trials in the UK. I like the taste and don't experience any side effects, but at the moment I still use erythritol, which is readily available and gives a pleasant, sweet flavour.

What you use to sweeten your food depends on how you feel about using artificial sweeteners. In the nutritional analysis after each recipe, you can see the differing values depending on the sweetener you use, so you can make informed choices. See our website, www.thegoodkitchentable.com, for more information on sweeteners and their pros and cons.

Terminology and what you will need

See pages 12–13 for what I mean when I refer to the following air fryer equipment in the recipes:

Crisper: or crisper plate

Drawer: also called a basket on some models

Rack: used to move food nearer the heat source

Baking paper liners

Reuseable silicone paper liner: cut to shape

Silicone liner

Little ovenproof dishes from charity shops, grandma's hand-me-downs, those ramekins at the back of the cupboard – all suddenly come in handy with an air fryer. I also reccomend the following, links to which can be found on our website, www.thegoodkitchentable.com:

Digital scales

Measuring spoons

Nonstick angled slice: for lifting out

Nonstick baking paper

Refillable oil spray with a good nozzle: I like a steel mister-style spray bottle

Silicone brush

Silicone muffin moulds

Silicone spatula

Silicone-tipped tongs: for picking up food

Small heatproof bowls, plates and dishes

Small oven gloves: I like silicone gloves

Temperature probe

Tin foil

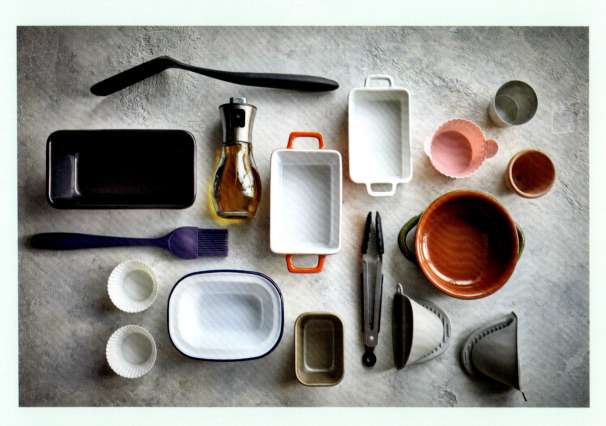

Drug-free Type 2 Diabetes Remission and Improving Your Health

Dr David Unwin, clinical expert in diabetes, Royal College of General Practitioners

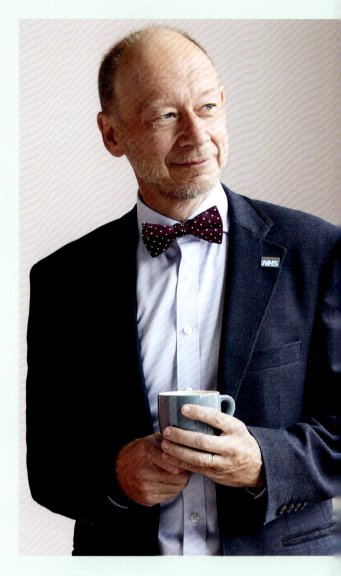

As a family doctor in the UK NHS, I have looked after the same population in the north of Liverpool since 1986. In that time, I have seen an astonishing ten-fold increase in the prevalence of type 2 diabetes and the metabolic problems like central obesity, high blood pressure and fatty liver that come with it. Something very similar has occurred in practices across the land and indeed around the world. A modern pandemic that means mine is the first generation ever who tragically enjoys a better life expectancy than our children. It's so bad that only one in ten boys born now can expect to reach retirement age in good health!

So how have we got into this mess?

A hint is given by a recent publication that looked at the diet of 3,000 UK adolescents. Junk food (more properly called ultra-processed food) accounted for 66 per cent of their total daily calories! Typically, ultra-processed food is made of cheap ingredients like sugar, refined carbohydrates and vegetable oils, often with a long shelf life to match its long list of ingredients. Sugar and refined carbohydrates like wheat flour are typically very calorific but nutrient depleted, leading to modern populations that are 'overfed but undernourished'. This helps explain why so many of my patients have a weight problem and yet at the same time are vitamin deficient. In fact, this phenomenon is rather more serious than that: recent studies have shown that those people consuming a high amount of ultra-processed foods have a 26 per cent increased risk of death from any cause. They were also more likely to develop type 2 diabetes and have poor mental health.

All of this makes it pretty clear we should be avoiding junk foods altogether, which is the point of this book. We want to show you how easy it is to use an air fryer to make healthy, nutrient-dense ingredients into delicious, affordable food.

Some of you will know that my passion is helping people with type 2 diabetes achieve drug-free remission by improving their diet, something we started in my practice back in 2013. So far, one-quarter of all my patients with type 2 diabetes have achieved remission by adopting a low-carb diet: 144 individuals to date. Our message is very simple: 'Just eat nutrient-dense food that doesn't put your blood sugar up.' After all, it is high blood sugars that over time shorten life and lead to the terrible side effects of diabetes. This means it makes sense to avoid not just sugar but also the starchy carbohydrates like rice, bread or potatoes that digest down into surprisingly large amounts of sugar. A good example is boiled white rice; a portion of just 150g (5½oz) (a small bowl) can be expected to raise your blood sugar to a similar extent as ten teaspoons of sugar! Even brown rice, at seven teaspoons of sugar, isn't much better.

It may also help to summarize the three common sources of sugar in our diet:

· Naturally sweet foods like honey, raisins or bananas

· Foods sweetened with table sugar like cakes, biscuits or many 'low-fat' foods

· Starchy carbohydrates that digest down into glucose like bread, potatoes or rice

Sugars and starches make up one of the 'big three' macronutrient groups: carbohydrates

Hence the 'low-carb diet', which involves reducing the carbs while increasing intake of the other two macronutrient groups: protein and healthy fats. The good news is there are plenty of delicious, healthy foods composed mainly of these two food groups. Here is a list of some of them: green veg, red meat, chicken, duck, fish, shellfish, full-fat dairy, eggs, mushrooms, nuts and berries. All ingredients you will see transformed into tasty meals by an air fryer and the recipes in this book.

In my early days on this diet, I wondered what effect decreasing the carbs while increasing dietary proteins and fats could have on health markers other than blood sugar. Some of my colleagues were quite worried, so we started collecting baseline and latest follow-up data of all the risk factors normally monitored in general practice. We have been doing this since 2013. The results are very interesting and the basis of about nine peer reviewed papers we have published. So far, the average time our patients have been on the low-carb diet is about three years. Over the years, we have found improvements in all measures of cardiovascular risk, suggesting this approach could also be of great interest to people without diabetes who are hoping to avoid health problems or just lose weight and belly fat.

Getting back to type 2 diabetes: what do we mean by remission?

The idea of drug-free remission of diabetes is fairly new. For most of my career as a doctor, this was a chronic condition that was expected to deteriorate over the years, gradually needing more and more drugs to control it. Certainly, I never met anyone who achieved remission in my first 25 years as a GP. Then in 2012 I met a lady with type 2 diabetes who had (quite without my help) achieved blood sugars in the non-diabetic range and come off her diabetes medication. Since then, drug-free remission of type 2 diabetes has become a beacon of hope that has spread around the world. It's possible that someone diagnosed with diabetes today could have dramatically better health in just a few months' time. In fact, in our practice, looking at people diagnosed with diabetes in the previous year who chose a low-carb diet, 73 per cent were found to achieve remission. The statistics are even better for people with prediabetes who try a low-carb diet: 93 per cent have a normal blood sugar a year later. As I mentioned earlier, overall, 50 per cent of our patients with diabetes find themselves in remission on this diet. Perhaps you are wondering what happens to the other 50 per cent? We looked at this in our 2023 paper published in BMJ Nutrition. After nearly three years on the diet, in addition to the 50 per cent in remission, a further 47 per cent had improved their diabetic control by lowering blood sugar. As a result, since 2018, our UK NHS practice has saved approximately £370,000 on the diabetes drug budget!

What about exercise?

There is a great deal of emphasis on using exercise to improve blood glucose. In a way, rightly so, as muscular activity uses up those pesky blood sugars to create movement. The drawback is that this process can make you hungrier. People who exercise eat more, so they may not lose weight. This is why the evidence is that exercise is great for so many health outcomes except weight loss. When thinking about exercise, please consider which forms of exercise suit you best. Not everyone wants to go to the gym; walking and gardening count too!

In addition to better blood sugar, we have documented significant improvements in:

· **Weight:** the average person lost 10kg (22 pounds)

· **Blood pressure**, so that many people were able to come off BP medication

· **Cholesterol** and other blood fats

· **Kidney function**

So, our low-carb approach can deliver far more than just better blood sugar!

The good news is that improving your diet can transform your health

What my team has done for hundreds of patients you may be able to replicate in your own home. Many of us choose our medical future by the dietary choices we make each day. I really hope you will use this book to improve not just your own health but also the health of those you love.

Disclaimer: the low-carb approach for people on prescribed medication
This book is not here to replace the individual advice given by your GP or practice nurse, which is based on your own specific case and medical history. In general, if you are on prescribed medication, please check any major dietary changes with your prescribing doctor.

Dr David Unwin's sugar infographics

FOOD ITEM	GLYCAEMIC INDEX	SERVING SIZE	HOW DOES EACH FOOD AFFECT BLOOD GLUCOSE COMPARED WITH ONE 4G TEASPOON OF TABLE SUGAR?
Basmati rice (white)	69	150g (5½oz)	10.1
Potato (white, boiled)	96	150g (5½oz)	9.1
French fries (baked)	64	150g (5½oz)	7.5
Spaghetti (white, boiled)	39	180g (6¼oz)	6.6
Sweetcorn (boiled)	60	80g (2¾oz)	4.0
Frozen peas (boiled)	51	80g (2¾oz)	1.3
Banana	62	120g (4¼oz)	5.7
Apple	39	120g (4¼oz)	2.3
Wholemeal bread (small slice)	74	30g (1oz)	3.0
Broccoli	15	80g (2¾oz)	0.2
Eggs	0	60g (2¼oz)	0

Other foods in the very low glycaemic range are chicken, oily fish, almonds, mushrooms, cheese.

Why We Overeat

Dr Jen Unwin, Clinical Health Psychologist

How we got hooked on junk food

In the last few decades, food manufacturers have invested heavily in understanding what makes food irresistible to us. They want us to love their products and become a regular customer after all. The Pulitzer Prize-winning investigative journalist, Michael Moss, took a deep dive into the world of the large food manufacturers in his 2022 book *Hooked* and what he found should be a worry to us all. Ultra-processed foods are full of cheap ingredients such as refined flours, sugars, salt and seed oils and added chemicals to extend their shelf life and improve their 'mouth feel'. Such products are barely foods at all, more a form of oral entertainment. We are now suffering the consequences on a global scale in terms of our physical and mental health. These foods offer very little nutrition for the body and brain. So how is it that a few giant food manufacturers and fast-food outlets have so easily hijacked our eating habits? Why do we continue to crave and seek out foods we know are harming us?

We are not so far away in evolutionary terms from having to hunt and forage all our food. We were, and are still, driven by strong survival urges to seek out food of any kind, particularly foods that would ensure fat gain in the autumn so that we could survive the lean, cold winter months. Some food scientists think we love 'crunchy' foods because the crunch signals freshness and foods that are safe to eat. We also love creamy foods probably because dairy and fats were excellent sources of calories. Nuts, fruits and honey would have been seasonal and scarce and it would have required great persistence to obtain them.

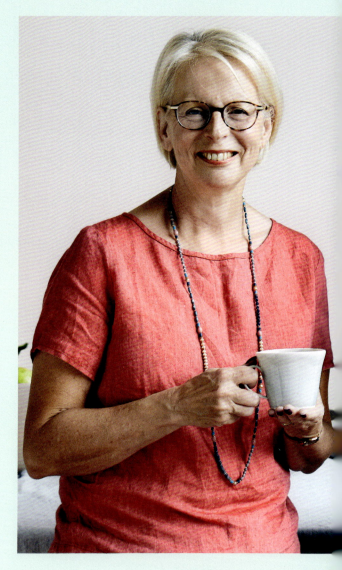

Junk food and your brain health

Our brains are highly attuned to seek out foods that are sweet, or that rare combination in nature of fat and carbohydrate. Nuts and dairy are the two main examples that many of us would find easy to overeat. Sweet foods or combinations of carbohydrate, salt and fat (doughnuts, pizza, fries...) lead to the release of unnaturally high levels of dopamine in the brain. Dopamine is the 'motivation and reward' messenger, and we feel temporarily good when it is available. The key word here is 'temporarily'. Like all things in the body, what goes up high must come down. Dopamine is the brain chemical largely responsible for all addictions; alcohol, nicotine, caffeine and drugs of abuse. We are driven to repeat the behaviour leading to the release of dopamine, however, each time the 'effect' is a little less, so we end up wanting more and more. Our brains are not designed to cope with the endless availability of ultra-processed foods and their impact on our neurotransmitters.

Every time we see an advert or walk down the crisp aisle in the supermarket, we are likely to experience cravings (as dopamine is released) and be drawn toward eating those foods. The part of the brain involved is easily tempted by advertising strategies: 'Just one won't hurt', 'I deserve a treat', and so on. We are overfed and undernourished. Researchers are now convinced of the harms that highly processed foods do to our physical and mental health and the part that their consumption is playing in the global epidemics of obesity, chronic disease and mental health problems.

How to escape the junk food trap

How can we train ourselves to eat differently and avoid the pull of sweet and processed foods? One strategy is to start focusing on eating real, whole foods that haven't been produced in a factory: cooking simple meals from scratch, like our ancestors. We all need time-saving ways of producing meals that will keep us healthy, and an air fryer is perfect for quick, delicious food that you know is doing you and your family good. I have seen many people escape the grip of addictive junk foods once they started to focus on real, whole foods as nature intended. Choosing to eat for nutrient density as opposed to entertainment is a massive step towards better health. Take the time to plan your meals and shopping list so that you are not tempted by processed options. Some people find it easier to shop online so they don't have to face the aisles of junk food. Treat your body and brain to real home-cooked food and soon you will start to notice improvements in energy, mood and sleep.

Air Fry Your Way To Health

Jenny Phillips, nutritionist and health coach
www.inspirednutrition.co.uk

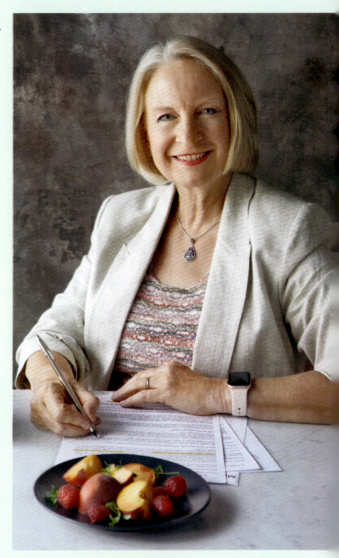

I, too, am an air fryer convert, having used one since 2019. It is a convenient addition to my empty nester kitchen, which is now mostly used to cook for two people. What makes this air fryer book different from others is that we are combining the health benefits of a low-carb diet with this way of cooking.

Low carb is an eating style based around foods that help to keep your blood sugars stable. Sugary and starchy foods, like rice, bread, pasta, pizza, potato crisps, biscuits and cake, quickly break down to sugar causing rapid rises in blood sugars. By restricting these foods and replacing them with delicious alternatives, you may be able to reverse prediabetes and type 2 diabetes or help to protect yourself from these conditions and keep yourself in good health.

So, what can you eat?

Let's think about the three macronutrients: protein, fat and carbohydrate (carbs).

Protein: good sources include meat, fish, dairy and eggs, plus the vegan proteins including nuts and seeds, pulses, beans, tofu and soy. Good-quality protein is needed for growth and repair; it also helps you to feel full and 'satiated'. I see many people in my nutrition practice who benefit enormously from increasing their protein intake.

Aim to include protein-rich foods in every meal and snack, to help build a strong and powerful body and to help prevent food cravings. Protein also helps to slow digestion and makes your blood sugar rise more slowly after meals.

Fats: these are the storage form of calories and hence are an excellent source of energy. Eating foods that contain fat, like meat, fish, nuts, cheese and avocados, and adding healthy fats (like olive oil) to your meals can help to keep your blood sugar levels steady. Healthy fats make food taste delicious and more satisfying, and as Dr Unwin's research shows, can help improve cardiovascular or heart health (see page 18).

We recommend cooking with extra-virgin olive oil, coconut oil, butter or animal fats like dripping – as Katie says (see page 14), keep it from your roasted meats and enjoy free food.

When you make your own treats, you can ensure that you use these good-quality fats in preference to the refined oils often used in industrially-produced food.

I don't recommend using vegetable oils or seed oils, like sunflower oil, for cooking. These oils are unstable when heated and prone to oxidation, which can then create inflammation in the body. Similarly, if you like to use an oil spray, consider purchasing an empty spray bottle and adding your own extra-virgin olive oil.

Carbs: provide energy and fibre for a healthy gut, but to maintain good blood sugar control, the type of carb matters. We use the CarbScale (see below) to help you to choose your carbohydrate intake to match your own situation. To start with, you may be unaware of 'where the carbs live', but with the nutrition information in this cookbook, plus reading food packet labels and maybe using a tracker app like Carbs & Cals or MyFitnessPal, you will soon be able to make better choices.

Starchy vegetables often grow underground and have more concentrated sugars. This group includes potatoes, sweet potatoes, butternut squashes, carrots, parsnips, beetroots, sweetcorn, turnips, etc.

Non-starchy vegetables include most other vegetables such as broccoli, cauliflower, green beans, aubergines, salad vegetables, avocados and many more.

For a more complete listing of the carb content of various foods, please visit our website: www.thegoodkitchentable.com.

How low should you go? Introducing the CarbScale

DIET	ARE YOU…	DAILY CARB TARGET
Keto	Prediabetic or type 2 diabetic?	30–50g
Strict low carb	Overweight?	50–75g
Moderate low carb	Healthy and want stable blood sugars?	75–100g
Liberal low carb	Fit, healthy and active and manage carbs well?	Up to 130g

How to use this book

Now that you're committed to trying the low-carb lifestyle by having purchased this cookbook, here are some tips to get you going:

1. Decide where you are on the CarbScale and choose your meals to match your carb intake. This stage is not forever, just until you know where excess carbs lie.

2. Find a food buddy. Having someone with whom you can discuss recipes and share experiences can be really motivational. Could you approach a family member, friend or colleague?

3. Build a store cupboard of commonly used ingredients (see page 14).

4. Set aside some time to read through the recipes and choose a couple to get started. Make a list of the ingredients you'll need and plan a time to try the recipes.

5. Reflect and build on your repertoire of foods. Ditch those that didn't work for you, and add those you liked to a short list. Rinse and repeat.

Is low carb expensive?

We often get push back from the media about cooking from scratch being too expensive, but is it really?

Yes, there are pricier options, such as steak, but even that can be relatively low in cost compared to, say, a takeaway, and steak is very quick and easy to cook. Also, you'll be cutting down on purchased treats, fizzy drinks and snacks, so there are potentially cost savings there.

If your budget is really tight, then consider recipes using these 'value for money' foods:

• Eggs

• Local, seasonal vegetables (these often cost less than imported, out of season varieties)

• Sardines and other canned fish

• Minced beef, lamb and pork

• Ungrated cheese (grate your own)

• Frozen vegetables, fish and meat

• Bulk packets of nuts and seeds

Budget-friendly recipes are marked with:

We really hope you enjoy aiming for your healthiest self with this low-carb cookbook, coupled with using your speedy and versatile air fryer.

Some Success Stories

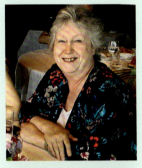

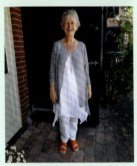

Elizabeth's Story

In 2017, after a lifetime of being overweight and yo-yo dieting, I was diagnosed with type 2 diabetes. I weighed 90kg (14 stone 2lbs) and had an HbA1C of 68. I thought I was already eating a 'healthy' diet, so my doctor prescribed medication.

However, I had heard that it was possible to put type 2 diabetes in remission by following a low carbohydrate lifestyle, so I decided to try that first before taking any medication. Three months later, my HbA1C was down to 35, and I had lost 19kg (3 stone) in weight! Seven years on, my diabetes remains in remission, and the weight has stayed off. And if I could do it, anyone can!

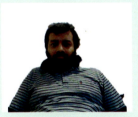

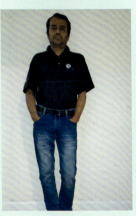

Shree's Story

I was diagnosed with type 2 diabetes in November 2023. My HbA1C result was an alarming 111, so my GP started insulin treatment at ten units a day. Three months later, my result was still quite high at 88. Despite the treatment, my blood glucose level was very erratic and never in range, so my dosage of insulin was increased to 18 units.

In January 2024, my GP offered me a TLC* course to help me learn more about type 2 diabetes and manage it better going forward. It was the best thing that has ever happened to me, as it gave me back control of my well-being and health. I immediately made changes to my eating habits by removing heavy carbs from my diet, and within a couple of weeks I could see my blood glucose level returning in range. I had to call my GP to stop the insulin as I no longer needed it.

In March 2024, my HbA1C was 47, and since then I have managed to maintain my blood glucose level within the normal range just by sticking to a low-carb diet.

*The Lifestyle Club (TLC) is an award-winning health coaching service for adults with Type 2 diabetes or prediabetes. You can find out more about TLC at www.thelifestyleclub.uk.

Meal Plans

To help you get started, we have created two meal plans. The first is perfect if you are the weight you want to be. However, many people diagnosed with type 2 diabetes may be advised to lose weight, and hence a weight loss plan is also included.

What do you notice? Yes, the meals are the same! If your goal is not to lose weight, you can enjoy healthy treats, too. We've even allowed for a glass or two of wine at the weekend. (This plan stays within the recommended limit of 14 units of alcohol per week.)

To lose weight, consistency is king. Stick to your healthy meals, don't snack in between and don't have any treats until your appetite and blood sugars are under control. You've got this!

● Breakfast   ● Lunch   ● Dinner

Weekly Meal Plan 1 – Weight Maintenance

	PROTEIN	CARBS	CALORIES
SATURDAY	**82**	**39**	**2139**
Mushroom Rarebit with 1 poached egg (see page 48)	19	3	338
1 Savoury Feta and Black Onion Seed Muffin (see page 171)	19	5	426
My Perfect Green Salad with Fresh Herbs and Vinaigrette (see page 200)	2	5	181
Fish with Tartare Sauce (see page 82)	30	3	420
Celeriac Fries (see page 141)	2	7	115
100g (3½oz) broccoli	2	4	35
2 x Stefano's Squidgy Chocolate, Date and Walnut Brownies (see page 191)	8	10	362
2 x 175ml (6fl oz) glasses of wine	0	2	262
SUNDAY	**93**	**68**	**2244**
The Full English – bacon, egg and tomato (see pages 38–43) and Sautéed Mushrooms (see page 150)	22	6	425
1 x Flowerpot bread roll (see page 157)	10	4	205
2 x Stefano's Squidgy Chocolate, Date and Walnut Brownies (see page 191), with 50g (1¾oz) mascarpone	10	12	576
Giancarlo's Tuscan Roast Chicken (see page 101)	36	0	394
Roasties (see page 140)	1	10	87
100g (3½oz) green beans	2	5	35
Blackberry and Apple Crumble (with erythritol) (see page 180)	7	21	273
175ml (6fl oz) glass of wine	0	1	131

	PROTEIN	CARBS	CALORIES
MONDAY	71	47	1434
Yogurt, Granola (see page 34) and Jammy Berry Compote (see page 33)	10	15	322
1 x Savoury Feta and Black Onion Seed Muffin (see page 171)	19	5	426
Sweetheart Cabbage and Carrot Slaw (see page 201)	2	5	105
Greek-inspired Chicken Salad with Halloumi Croutons (see page 104)	39	9	525
1 apple	1	13	56
TUESDAY	87	37	1581
1 x Breakfast Sausage Muffin (see page 44)	27	6	430
Curried Vegetable Soup with Crispy Paneer Croutons (see page 64)	15	16	495
1 x leftover Flowerpot bread roll (see page 157)	10	4	205
Crispy Duck, Pancetta and Blackberry Salad (see page 107)	32	6	334
3 x Mini Hazelnut and Chocolate Bites (see page 182)	3	5	117
WEDNESDAY	78	57	1608
Yogurt, Granola (see page 34) and Jammy Berry Compote (see page 33)	10	15	322
1 x Scotch Egg (see page 59)	33	3	518
Leftover Sweetheart Cabbage and Carrot Slaw (see page 201)	2	5	105
Sausages, Mash and Onion Gravy (see page 118)	26	10	523
100g (3½oz) frozen peas	6	11	84
1 apple	1	13	56
THURSDAY	112	46	1820
1 x Breakfast Sausage Muffin (see page 44)	27	6	430
Halloumi and Vegetable Skewers with Giorgio's Chilli Sauce (see page 129)	24	13	511
3 x Mini Hazelnut and Chocolate Bites (see page 182)	3	5	117
Narinder's Chicken Tikka (see page 103)	42	5	286
Cauliflower Rice (see page 199)	2	4	52
Cucumber Raita (see page 195)	2	2	54
Roast Strawberries and Lime Cheesecake Cream with Crumble (see page 184)	12	11	370
FRIDAY	105	58	1829
Yogurt, Granola (see page 34) and Jammy Berry Compote (see page 33)	10	15	322
Berber-style Omelette (see page 60)	15	18	316
Simple Steak with Garlic and Rosemary Butter (see page 108)	66	1	462
Roasted Mediterranean Vegetables (see page 138)	2	11	97
Roast Strawberries and Lime Cheesecake Cream with Crumble (see page 184)	12	11	370
2 x 175ml (6fl oz) glasses of wine	0	2	262

Weekly Meal Plan 2 – Weight Loss

	PROTEIN	CARBS	CALORIES
SATURDAY	**74**	**27**	**1515**
Mushroom Rarebit with 1 poached egg (see page 48)	19	3	338
1 x Savoury Feta and Black Onion Seed Muffin (see page 171)	19	5	426
My Perfect Green Salad with Fresh Herbs and Vinaigrette (see page 200)	2	5	181
Fish with Tartare Sauce (see page 82)	30	3	420
Celeriac Fries (see page 141)	2	7	115
100g (3½oz) broccoli	2	4	35
SUNDAY	**81**	**37**	**1722**
The Full English – bacon, egg and tomato (see pages 38–43) and Sautéed Mushrooms (see page 150)	22	6	425
1 x Flowerpot bread roll (see page 157)	10	4	205
2 x Stefano's Squidgy Chocolate, Date and Walnut Brownies (see page 191), with 50g (1¾oz) mascarpone	10	12	576
Giancarlo's Tuscan Roast Chicken (see page 101)	36	0	394
Roasties (see page 140)	1	10	87
100g (3½oz) green beans	2	5	35
MONDAY	**71**	**47**	**1434**
Yogurt, Granola (see page 34) and Jammy Berry Compote (see page 33)	10	15	322
1 x Feta and Black Onion Seed Muffin (see page 171)	19	5	426
Sweetheart Cabbage and Carrot Slaw (see page 201)	2	5	105
Greek-inspired Chicken Salad with Halloumi Croutons (see page 104)	39	9	525
1 apple	1	13	56
TUESDAY	**84**	**32**	**1464**
1 x Breakfast Sausage Muffin (see page 44)	27	6	430
Curried Vegetable Soup with Crispy Paneer Croutons (see page 64)	15	16	495
1 x leftover Flowerpot bread roll (see page 157)	10	4	205
Crispy Duck, Pancetta and Blackberry Salad (see page 107)	32	6	334

The Diabetes Air Fryer Cookbook

	PROTEIN	CARBS	CALORIES
WEDNESDAY	**77**	**44**	**1552**
Yogurt, Granola (see page 34) and Jammy Berry Compote (see page 33)	10	15	322
1 x Scotch Egg (see page 59)	33	3	518
Leftover Sweetheart Cabbage and Carrot Slaw (see page 201)	2	5	105
Sausages, Mash and Onion Gravy (see page 118)	26	10	523
100g (3½oz) frozen peas	6	11	84
THURSDAY	**97**	**30**	**1333**
1 x Breakfast Sausage Muffin (see page 44)	27	6	430
Halloumi and Vegetable Skewers with Giorgio's Chilli Sauce (see page 129)	24	13	511
Narinder's Chicken Tikka (see page 103)	42	5	286
Cauliflower Rice (see page 199)	2	4	52
Cucumber Raita (see page 195)	2	2	54
FRIDAY	**93**	**45**	**1197**
Yogurt, Granola (see page 34) and Jammy Berry Compote (see page 33)	10	15	322
Berber-style Omelette (see page 60)	15	18	316
Simple Steak with Garlic and Rosemary Butter (see page 108)	66	1	462
Roasted Mediterranean Vegetables (see page 138)	2	11	97

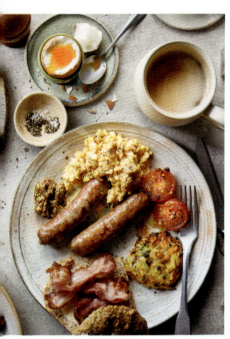
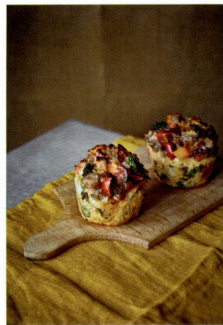
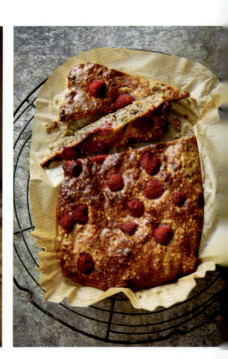

BREAKFAST

A Note on Breakfast

How can breakfast be the most important meal of the day but it's fine to skip it? It was Dr Kellogg, of the cereal fame, who promoted breakfast as an important meal. However, when you follow a low-carb lifestyle, the gnawing hunger of a carb-heavy diet often disappears; there's no point eating if you're trying to lose weight and aren't hungry (unless there are medical reasons).

If you are having breakfast, start the day with a savoury one or one with minimal sugar, otherwise you may find yourself kicking off those glucose swings, getting sleepy or hungry mid-morning and reaching for the biscuit tin. The air fryer gives you plenty of quick and easy breakfast options.

Good choices are eggs, our low-carb bakes, full-fat Greek yogurt or homemade granola. They are low in carbs and high in protein to keep you fuller for longer. Poor choices are sugary cereals, pastries and sweet milky drinks or fruit juice. Here are a few examples of typical breakfast choices:

	NET CARBS	PROTEIN
1 cup (215g/7½oz) of fruit smoothie (no dairy)	25g	1g
250ml (9fl oz) glass of freshly squeezed orange juice	25g	2g
100g (3½oz) Scottish porridge oats	60g	10g
30g (1oz) Special K Original	22g	5g
1 thick slice (40g/1½oz) of granary bread	18g	4g
1 thick slice (40g/1½oz) of organic sourdough bread	20g	2g
20g (¾oz) good-quality marmalade	13g	0.1g
1 banana	17g	1g
1 grande (225ml/8fl oz) caffè latte with flavoured syrup	21g	6g
1 medium (225ml/8fl oz) americano	0g	0g
30ml (1fl oz) double cream	0g	0g
30ml (1fl oz) full-fat milk	1g	1g
30g (1oz) walnuts	2g	5g
100g (3½oz) 10%-fat Greek yogurt	5g	6g
75g (2½oz) raspberries	4g	1g
2 large boiled or poached eggs	1g	13g
2 milk chocolate digestives	21g	2g

Jammy Berry Compote

Serves 10
(makes approx.
350g/12oz)

By making a jammy compote from berries, you can keep the carbs down, as very little sweetness is needed. I make this quickly by using inexpensive frozen misshapen berries straight from the freezer (available in most supermarkets) in winter or fresh berries in summer. Use any berries you have: all one type or a mixture.

1. Put the berries, vanilla, sweetener, if using, and any flavourings into the empty drawer, or use a silicone liner or ovenproof dish.

2. Air fry at 200°C (400°F) for 6 minutes, or until the berries are soft, shaking halfway through. Roughly mash the berries, particularly any large strawberries, to create a jammy consistency. If the compote is very watery, put it back in and cook for a couple more minutes.

3. Tip the berries into a bowl or container and allow to cool. Serve straight away or decant into jars when it is room temperature. Store in the refrigerator for up to week. The jam can also be frozen for up to 3 months.

400g (14oz) frozen blueberries,
    raspberries, blackberries,
    strawberries, blackcurrants
    or redcurrants
2 teaspoons vanilla extract
2 teaspoons erythritol or honey
    (optional)
flavourings of your choice (optional,
    see below)

Tips and tricks
Flavour the jam: add a couple of pieces of orange or lemon peel and/or a star anise.

Fresh berries: if using these, reduce the cooking time by approximately half.

Per serving (approx. 35g/1¼oz) with erythritol: 22kcal			
NET CARBS	FIBRE	PROTEIN	FAT
4g	1g	0g	0g

Per serving (approx. 35g/1¼oz) with honey: 26kcal			
NET CARBS	FIBRE	PROTEIN	FAT
6g	1g	0g	0g

Granola

Nuts are great for filling us up, providing insoluble fibre for our gut health, and providing vitamins and healthy fats. This recipe makes a large amount, which is ideal to store in a jar so you can measure out portions as you need. Making your own granola is much better than buying the sugar-laden ones in the shops. Even if they don't contain added sugar, they often have raisins or dates in the mix. If you don't have time for breakfast, take a serving of the dry granola to work and have it with a coffee. Otherwise, top Greek yogurt with the granola, add a few berries or Jammy Berry Compote (see page 33), and finish with some finely grated orange zest. To weigh out the honey, hold a spoon in hot water briefly before spooning it out, so it will easily slip off.

1. Melt the butter and honey together in a small heatproof bowl in the air fryer or a microwave.

2. Put the remaining ingredients in a larger bowl, pour in the melted butter and honey, then stir thoroughly.

3. Spread out the mixture on a crisper in the drawer, or use a silicone liner or ovenproof dish. If you use a crisper, this will help ensure the granola is crunchy; if the seeds fall through, you can pick them up later after baking.

4. Bake the granola at 200°C (400°F) for 7–8 minutes until browned and dry, tossing gently with a spatula every 2 minutes to ensure even browning.

5. Tip the granola on to a plate and allow it to cool. It can be stored in a jar at room temperature for up to 4 days or in the refrigerator for up to a week.

25g (1oz) unsalted butter
    or coconut oil
20g (¾oz) honey or erythritol
1 egg white, lightly beaten
150g (5½oz) mixed nuts (such as
    almonds, hazelnuts, walnuts
    and pecans)
75g (2½oz) mixed seeds (pumpkin,
    flax, sunflower, sesame)
2 teaspoons vanilla extract
2 teaspoons ground cinnamon
finely grated zest of 1 small orange

Per serving (approx. 35g/1¼oz) with honey: 169kcal			
NET CARBS	FIBRE	PROTEIN	FAT
4g	2g	4g	15g
Per serving (approx. 35g/1¼oz) with erythritol: 163kcal			
NET CARBS	FIBRE	PROTEIN	FAT
2g	2g	4g	15g

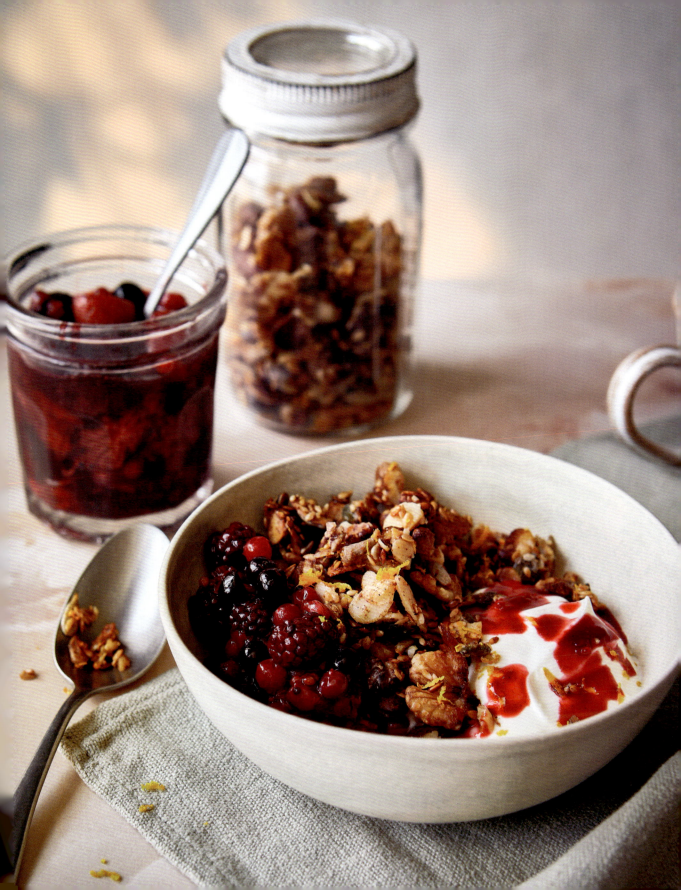

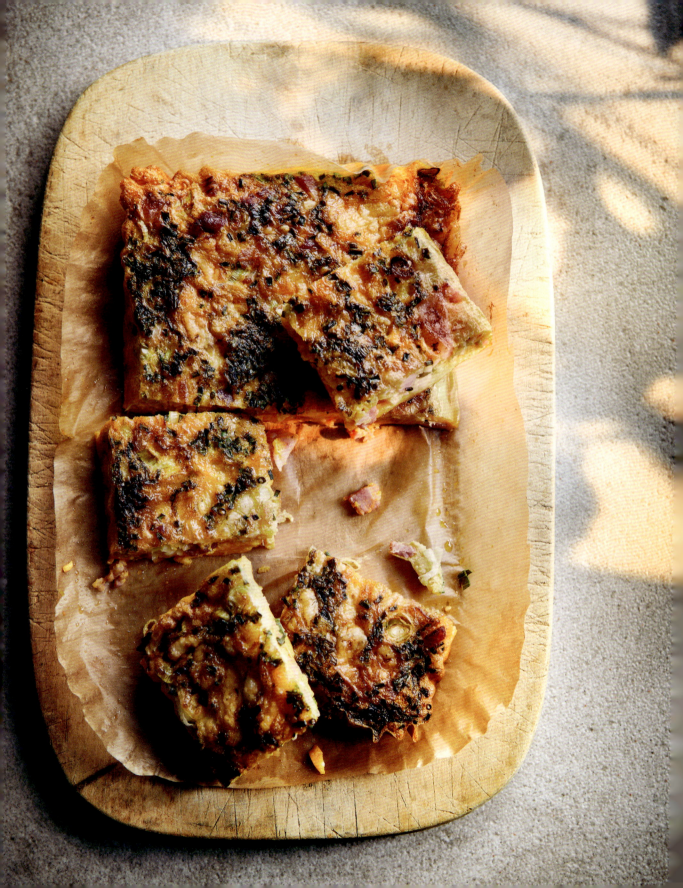

Bacon, Spring Onion and Smoked Cheese Frittata

This is an ideal breakfast or lunch. Use the cooking time to get ready for the day or to make a salad to go with it. Alter the ingredients to use up what's in the refrigerator: leave out the bacon and use roast red peppers instead, and change the cheese to your favourite.

1. Put the bacon, spring onions and oil in a trimmed baking paper liner in a silicone liner or ovenproof dish, season and then place in the drawer. Cook at 200°C (400°F) for 3–5 minutes until lightly browned.

2. Beat the eggs in a mixing bowl and stir in the cheese and herbs, if using.

3. Pull out the drawer, leaving the dish inside. Make sure the bacon and onions are evenly distributed over the base of the dish and then pour in the eggs.

4. Return the drawer and then bake at 160°C (325°F) for 15 minutes, or until browned and cooked through underneath. You can check this by making a cut in the top with a knife. Have a peek inside and see if it is runny underneath; if it is, cover with tin foil tucked into the sides and cook it for a few more minutes.

5. Serve in the paper liner or the dish. Serve on its own or with tomatoes or salad.

4 bacon streaky rashers, chopped, or lardons (120g/4¼oz)
4 spring onions or ½ small onion, finely chopped
1 tablespoon extra-virgin olive oil
4 eggs
25g (1oz) smoked Cheddar or other hard cheese, coarsely grated
handful of chopped herbs, such as chives or parsley (optional)
salt and pepper

Per serving: 388kcal			
NET CARBS	FIBRE	PROTEIN	FAT
3g	1g	25g	31g

The Full English (pictured overleaf)

Air fryers are great for cooked breakfasts for one or two. With the use of a rack, you can double the space and have crispy bacon cooking over tomatoes or a fried egg. I love to do this as the bacon fat drips down on to the food underneath, so it's a win, win! Slow the cooking of some foods down such as tomatoes, mushrooms or fried eggs by placing them on the bottom of the drawer or in a silicone liner, or speed things up like bacon or grilled tomatoes by putting them on the rack. Here are a few suggestions of different elements which you can use to build your perfect breakfast or brunch. For extra sides that go well with this dish, see the Sautéed Mushrooms on page 150 or the Cheesy Vegetable Hash Browns opposite.

Bacon
Place 3 streaky bacon rashers on a high rack and air fry at 200°C (400°F) for 5–7 minutes. Alternatively, place the bacon on a crisper at the base of the drawer and air fry for around 7 minutes. If the air can circulate easily, I find I don't need to turn the rashers (you may need to turn them halfway through the cooking time if using the crisper).

Per 3 streaky bacon rashers (70g/2½oz): 190kcal			
NET CARBS	FIBRE	PROTEIN	FAT
0g	0g	10g	17g

Halloumi Cheese Slices
Halloumi makes a great veggie alternative in a fry-up. Place 2 x 40g (1½oz) halloumi slices (1cm- (½ inch)-thick) on an oiled rack or crisper in the drawer and air fry at 200°C (400°F) for 6–8 minutes.

Per 40g (1½oz) slice: 130kcal			
NET CARBS	FIBRE	PROTEIN	FAT
1g	0g	8g	10g

Sausages
Choose high-meat-content sausages to lower the carbs. Put 2 sausages in a single layer on a crisper and air fry at 180°C (350°F) for 10–15 minutes, turning once, until they are browned and done. To check, cut a sausage and make sure it isn't pink inside.

Per 2 sausages: 340kcal			
NET CARBS	FIBRE	PROTEIN	FAT
0g	0g	23g	28g

Frozen Sausages
Air fry the frozen sausages (separately or frozen together) on a rack at 180°C (350°F) for 5 minutes to defrost. Spread them out on the rack and continue to cook at 180°C (350°F) for 10–15 minutes, turning once halfway through.

Per 2 sausages: 340kcal			
NET CARBS	FIBRE	PROTEIN	FAT
0g	0g	23g	28g

Grilled Tomatoes
Thickly slice a small tomato and place the slices into the drawer under a rack. Season with salt and pepper and spray with ½ teaspoon of oil. Air fry at 200°C (400°F) for 10–12 minutes or 4–6 minutes if using a high rack.

Per 80g (2¾oz) tomato with oil: 34kcal			
NET CARBS	FIBRE	PROTEIN	FAT
2g	1g	1g	2g

Cheesy Vegetable Hash Browns

(pictured overleaf)

Enjoy these with eggs or bacon for breakfast, or take them to work with a dip and a boiled egg for extra protein. Halve the recipe for a small batch or freeze some for another day. Use any hard cheese you have in your refrigerator or a mixture of odds and ends.

1. Line a crisper with nonstick baking paper.

2. Boil 1.7 litres (3 pints) water. Meanwhile, coarsely grate the root vegetables in a food processor or by hand. Put them into a bowl and pour over the boiling water to cover. Stir and then leave to stand for 5 minutes, stirring a couple of times.

3. Tip the vegetables into a colander and press the bottom of the empty bowl into the colander to drain them well. Set aside to cool for a few minutes.

4. In a large mixing bowl, stir together the egg, shallot, flour, cheese, herbs, salt and plenty of pepper. Add the vegetables and stir through to combine. Divide the mixture into 50g (1¾oz) balls and squeeze them gently with your hands to form them into burger shapes, discarding any liquid.

5. Lay them on the lined crisper in the drawer and air fry at 200°C (400°F) for 5 minutes until just firm to the touch. Use a spatula to turn them over to the other side and return to the air fryer for another 4 minutes or until golden brown.

6. Serve hot or at room temperature. They will keep for up to 3 days in an airtight container in the refrigerator or up to 3 months, tightly wrapped, in the freezer.

Tips and tricks
Alter the flavour by adding a heaped teaspoon of spice such as smoked paprika, ground cumin, ras el hanout or black onion (nigella) seeds.

225g (8oz) trimmed and peeled root vegetables (such as swede, celeriac, carrot, turnip, sweet potato)
1 egg
50g (1¾oz) shallot, leek, onion or spring onions, finely chopped
25g (1oz) chickpea flour
50g (1¾oz) smoked or mature Cheddar, halloumi or firm mozzarella cheese, finely grated
7g (¼oz) fresh chives, parsley or coriander, finely chopped, or 1 teaspoon dried thyme or oregano
½–1 teaspoon salt (depending on your cheese)
freshly ground black pepper

Per serving of 2 hash browns: 134kcal			
NET CARBS	FIBRE	PROTEIN	FAT
9g	2g	7g	7g

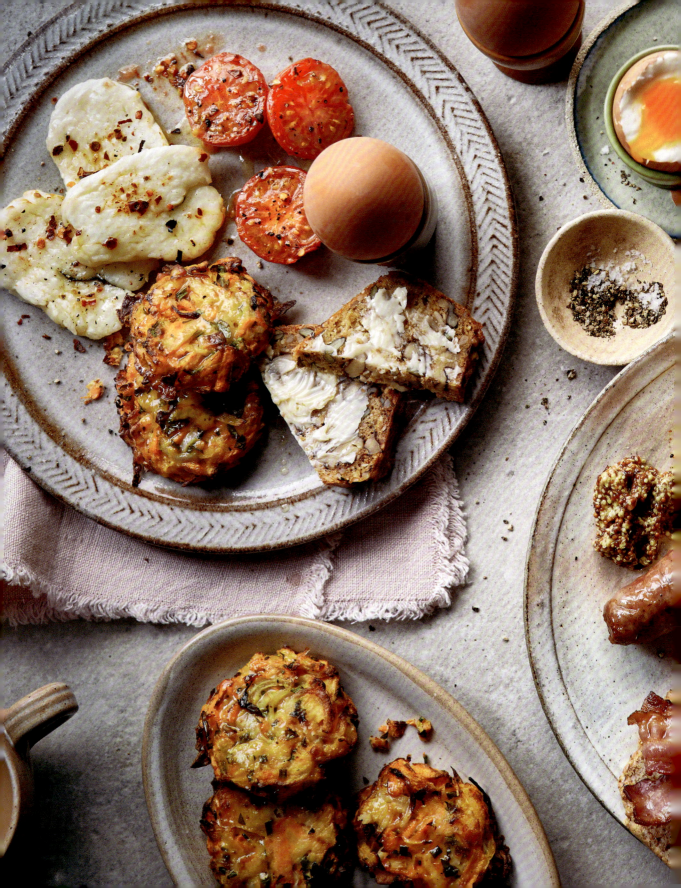

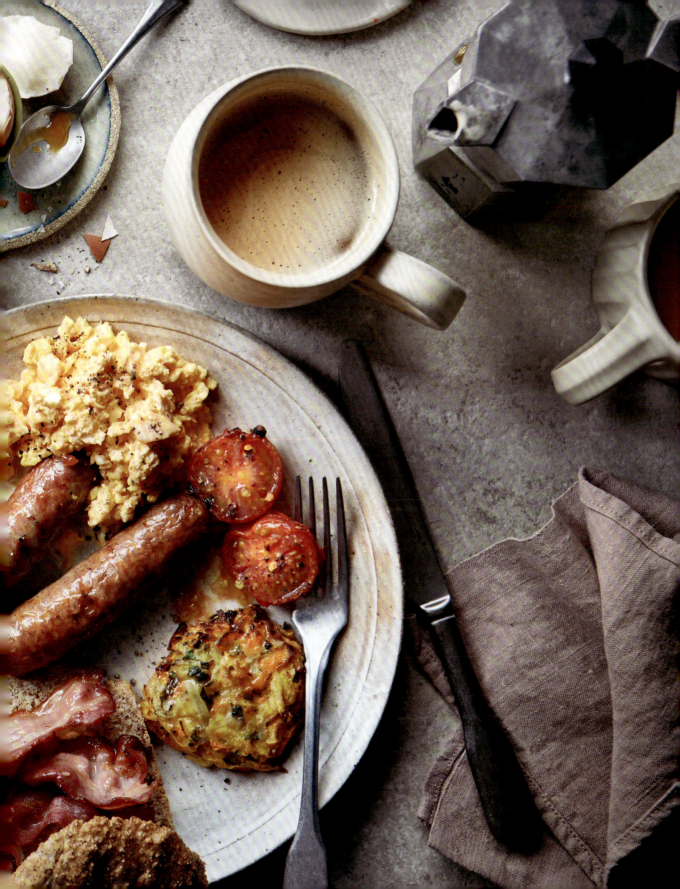

Eggs

Eggs are just perfect for breakfast when you are following a low-carb lifestyle. They are rich in protein, quick and easy to cook, and have almost no carbs.

Air fryers make hot, dry heat, which can easily overcook yolks and undercook whites. There are loads of recipes online for how to poach or bake whole eggs in an air fryer, but I think nothing beats a pan of water or a slow oven when you need to see what's going on. However, fried, scrambled, boiled and frittata-style are excellent made in an air fryer.

Scrambled Eggs (pictured on pages 40–41)

With a small, ovenproof dish, you can have creamy scrambled eggs in less than 5 minutes without the eggy frying pan that's hard to wash. My tip is to use the same dish each time, so that you will learn the exact timing with practice. Add 50g (1¾oz) smoked or cooked salmon, a slice of grilled halloumi, one of the low-carb breads (see page 156) or a couple of bacon rashers to bump up the protein. Stir in 1 tablespoon of chopped herbs at step 2, such as celery leaves, dill or parsley, for extra flavour.

1. Heat a small ovenproof dish on a crisper in the drawer of your air fryer at 200°C (400°F) for 3 minutes.

2. Meanwhile, in a jug, beat the eggs together with the crème fraiche and seasoning.

3. When the dish is warm, remove the drawer, leaving the dish in the drawer, and use a knife (or a heatproof silicone brush) to wipe the butter around the warm dish – it will melt on contact. Tilt the drawer to ensure the butter covers the base of the dish. Now pour the egg mixture into the dish, using a silicone spatula to help.

4. Air fry the eggs for 3 minutes. Remove the drawer, then stir the eggs with the spatula, combining the set edges with the soft inside. Replace the drawer and continue to cook for 30 seconds more, or until set around the edges again.

5. Remove the drawer and use tongs, an angled slice or oven gloves to remove the hot dish. Stir the eggs in the dish and use the residual heat to cook them to your liking. Eat from the container with any toppings or tip the eggs on to a plate with the help of the spatula and enjoy.

2 eggs
1 tablespoon crème fraîche
  or double cream
10g (¼oz) butter
small pinch of salt
freshly ground black pepper

Per serving of scrambled eggs: 257kcal			
NET CARBS	FIBRE	PROTEIN	FAT
1g	0g	12g	23g
Per serving with smoked or cooked salmon: 338kcal			
NET CARBS	FIBRE	PROTEIN	FAT
2g	0g	23g	26g

Fried Eggs

This is just a guide, as I don't know the size of your eggs
or containers or how you like your eggs in the morning!

1. Spray oil (or use melted bacon fat or dripping) over the drawer or
    into a silicone liner or ovenproof container on a crisper. Crack your
    egg(s) into the container and air fry at 180°C (350°F) for 5 minutes.
    If other foods are on a rack above, allow 6 minutes.

Per fried egg in ½ teaspoon oil: 88kcal			
NET CARBS	FIBRE	PROTEIN	FAT
0.5g	0g	6g	7g

Boiled Eggs (pictured on pages 40–41)

The more you boil eggs in your own air fryer, the more confident
you will be about the time it takes to cook your perfect egg.

1. Preheat the air fryer to 130°C (265°F) with a crisper in the drawer.

2. Put the eggs on the crisper. For soft-boiled eggs: air fry medium
    eggs for 11 minutes and large eggs for 12 minutes. For hard-boiled
    eggs: air fry medium or large eggs for 15 minutes.

3. Eat straight away or plunge into cold water and crack the shells
    to stop blue rings from forming. Roll the eggs on a flat surface to
    crack the shells all around. Carefully peel off the shells and use
    straight away or store in a container in the refrigerator for up to
    2 days.

Per boiled egg: 68kcal			
NET CARBS	FIBRE	PROTEIN	FAT
0.5g	0g	6g	5g

Breakfast Sausage Muffins

Use any leftover vegetables that you have in the refrigerator instead of the list below. This is based on an American breakfast casserole often baked in cake tins and cut into wedges. I like to make mine in muffin moulds, as they cook quickly and come out easily, so are perfect for taking to work for breakfast or lunch. If you are keeping your carbs very low, substitute the squash for cooked and well-squeezed spinach instead.

1. You will need 2 silicone muffin moulds, approx. 8cm (3¼ inches) diameter, 4.5cm (1¾ inches) deep.

2. Score a line down the sausages, and peel away the skins. Crumble the sausagemeat from the cases into the drawer of your air fryer. Add the peppers, butternut squash or spinach, spring onions, broccoli, chilli, oregano, if using, and oil and stir through using a silicone spatula. Air fry the mixture at 200°C (400°F) for 7–10 minutes until soft and lightly browned and any water has evaporated.

3. Meanwhile, beat the eggs in a mixing bowl and add the cheese.

4. Now tip the vegetable and sausage mixture into the bowl and mix well with the eggs. Use a spoon to divide the mixture between the 2 moulds and then air fry at 160°C (325°F) for 5 minutes, or until firm to the touch.

5. Remove the muffins from the drawer and set aside for 5 minutes before turning out of the moulds. Serve straight away or allow to cool. They will keep for up to 3 days in the refrigerator or up to 3 months in the freezer.

3 high-meat-content sausages
75g (2½oz) frozen or fresh red peppers, chopped
75g (2½oz) cubed butternut squash or cooked and squeezed spinach
2 spring onions, roughly chopped
75g (2½oz) frozen or fresh broccoli florets
pinch of chilli flakes or a little chopped fresh hot chilli
1 teaspoon dried oregano (optional)
2 teaspoons extra-virgin olive oil
2 eggs
15g (½oz) Cheddar, smoked Cheddar or other firm cheese, coarsely grated
salt and pepper

Per muffin with squash: 430kcal			
NET CARBS	FIBRE	PROTEIN	FAT
6g	3g	27g	33g
Per muffin with spinach: 423kcal			
NET CARBS	FIBRE	PROTEIN	FAT
4g	3g	27g	33g

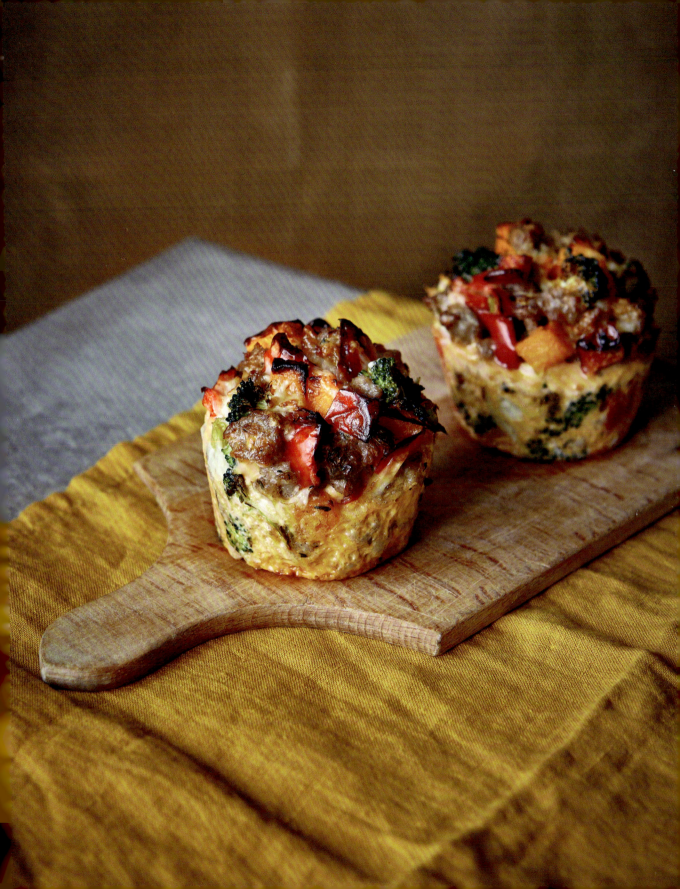

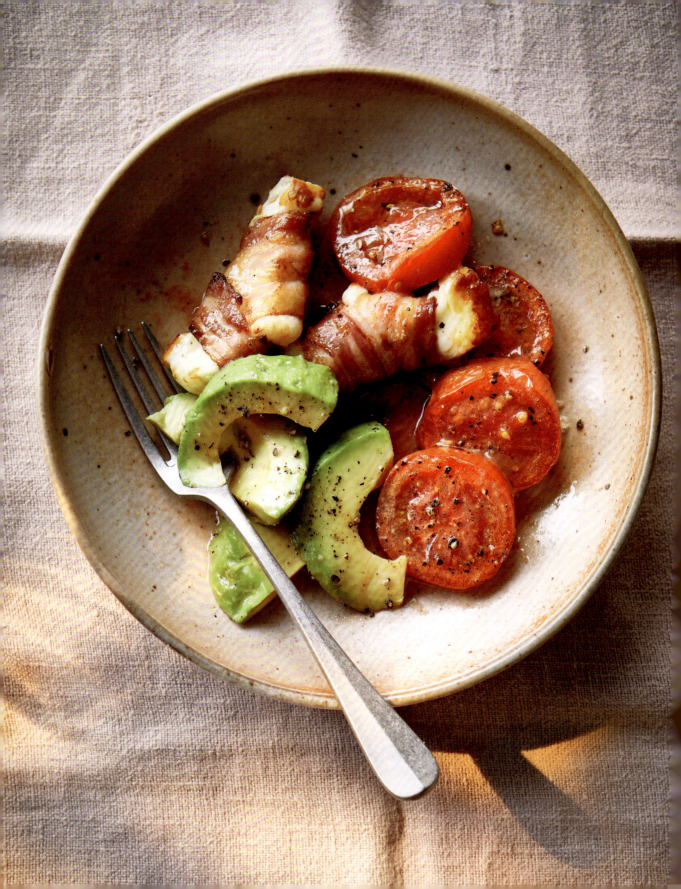

Halloumi Wrapped in Bacon
with Avocado and Grilled Tomatoes

This gorgeous, colourful breakfast or brunch can be cooked at the
same time in the air fryer. If time is short, pre-wrap the halloumi
the night before and leave, covered, in the refrigerator. If you are
cooking this for one, preserve half the avocado in the refrigerator by
replacing the stone and covering it with the skin of the sliced half.

1. Spray or brush the oil over the base of the air fryer drawer or an
   ovenproof container. Lay the cherry tomato halves over the oil,
   give the tops another spray and evenly season them with pepper
   and a little salt. Put a rack over the top.

2. Wrap each slice of halloumi with a bacon rasher. Lay these on the
   rack. Air fry at 200°C (400°F) for 7–9 minutes, or until browned and
   starting to crisp. Have a look at the bacon underneath: usually it
   doesn't need further cooking, as the air has circulated under the
   rack. If it looks underdone, turn each halloumi slice and give them
   another 2 minutes.

3. Meanwhile, arrange the avocado slices on 2 plates.

4. When the halloumi slices are done, add them to the plates,
   followed by the tomatoes. Serve straight away.

1 teaspoon extra-virgin olive oil,
  plus extra for spraying
4 cherry tomatoes, halved
125g (4½oz) halloumi cheese, cut into
  4 slices around 1cm (½ inch) wide
4 rashers smoked or unsmoked
  streaky bacon
flesh of 1 ripe avocado, sliced
salt and pepper

Per serving: 433kcal			
NET CARBS	FIBRE	PROTEIN	FAT
5g	3g	20g	37g

Mushroom Rarebit

I love using big field mushrooms for this recipe, which makes an easy brunch or a light supper. Serve on its own, with the Creamy Spinach with Nutmeg on page 151 or a couple of tomatoes on the side. To add protein, enjoy it with any of the egg recipes on pages 42–43.

1. Use a small knife to cut away the stalks of the mushrooms; set aside the stalks. Lay the mushrooms, gill-side up, on a silicone liner or an ovenproof dish. Brush with the oil and season with salt and pepper. Place in the air fryer drawer and air fry at 200°C (400°F) for 3 minutes, or until tender and darker around the edges. Using tongs, turn the mushrooms over so the domed sides are facing upward and grill for 2 minutes.

2. Meanwhile, make the filling. Finely chop the mushroom stalks and then mix them with all the remaining ingredients in a bowl using a fork or whisk.

3. Remove the mushrooms from the air fryer. Turn them gill-side up again. Spoon the filling into their cavities. Air fry for another 4–6 minutes, or until golden brown. Any extra filling can be cooked in a small ramekin or egg cup at the same time. Serve warm.

2 large portobello mushrooms (150g/5½oz), brushed clean
1 teaspoon extra-virgin olive oil
1 egg
25g (1oz) mature Cheddar or other hard cheese, coarsely grated
½ teaspoon Dijon mustard
couple of drops of Worcestershire sauce (optional, leave this out if you don't eat fish)
1 tablespoon Greek yogurt, crème fraîche or double cream
salt and pepper

Per serving: 270kcal			
NET CARBS	FIBRE	PROTEIN	FAT
2g	2g	13g	23g

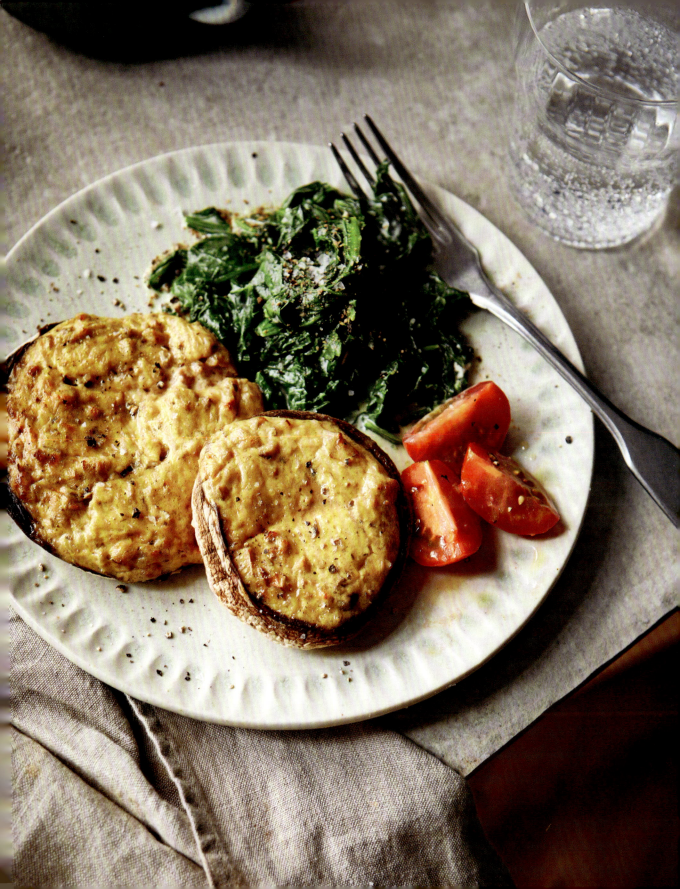

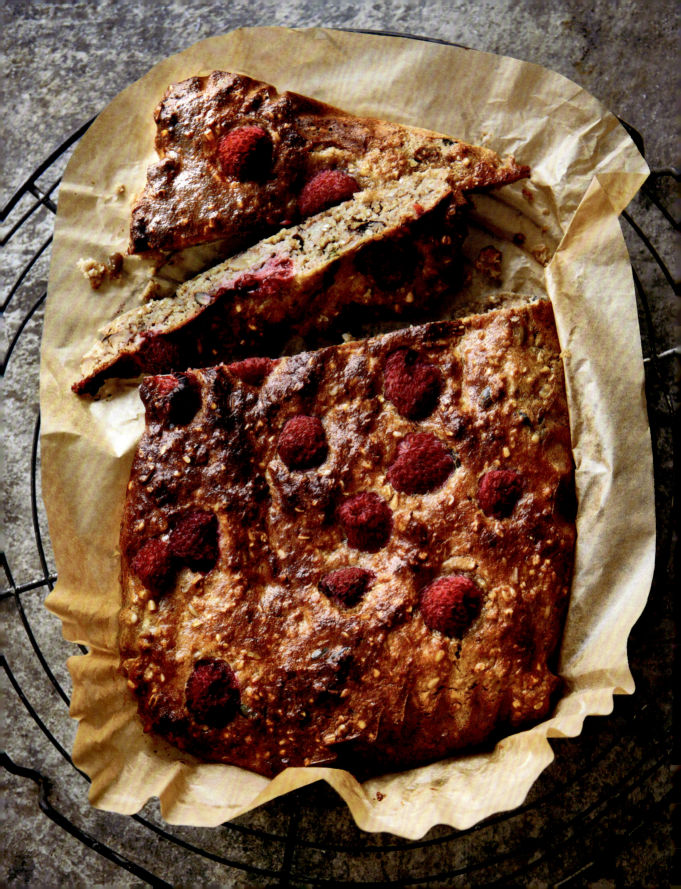

Baked Oats with Seeds and Walnuts

Although 'baked oats' have recently experienced a resurgence, the delicious and filling dish of set porridge is also a blast from the past. Our Glaswegian friend Brian McLeod told me about his mother's porridge that was poured into a drawer where it set firm. She sliced pieces off to feed her children who were about to run to school and needed energy.

A 40g (1½oz) serving of porridge made with water typically contains 24g net carbs. Since most of us don't immediately run after breakfast, this can give us a large spike in glucose levels, so in this recipe, I have replaced most of the oats with nuts and seeds to lower the carbs.

Flavour the loaf with cinnamon, orange zest or mixed spices as you wish, or leave them out altogether. The mixture can also be cooked in 6 silicone muffin moulds. You may find the sweetness of the banana enough to omit the sweeteners. I like to eat a square of this with thick Greek yogurt.

1. Mash the banana with a fork in a mixing bowl, then add the remaining ingredients except the berries.

2. Put a baking paper liner or an ovenproof dish into the drawer. Spoon the mixture into the liner or dish and flatten it out a little with the back of the spoon. Evenly scatter over the berries. Bake at 160°C (325°F) for 16 minutes, or until a skewer poked into the middle comes out clean.

3. Leave in the warmth of the drawer to cool and set firm. Once cooled, wrap and keep in the refrigerator for up to 3 days.

1 small banana (approx. 110g/3¾oz), roughly chopped
35g (1¼oz) steel-cut porridge oats
75g (2½oz) ground almonds
35g (1¼oz) mixed chopped nuts
2 eggs
25g (1oz) seeds such as sunflower, linseed or pumpkin
2 teaspoons vanilla extract
2 tablespoons erythritol or 4 teaspoons honey (optional)
1 teaspoon ground cinnamon or mixed spice or ½ teaspoon finely grated orange zest
½ teaspoon baking powder
pinch of salt
50g (1¾oz) raspberries or other berries, fresh or frozen

Per serving with erythritol: 201kcal			
NET CARBS	FIBRE	PROTEIN	FAT
10g	3g	7g	14g
Per serving with honey: 215kcal			
NET CARBS	FIBRE	PROTEIN	FAT
14g	3g	7g	14g

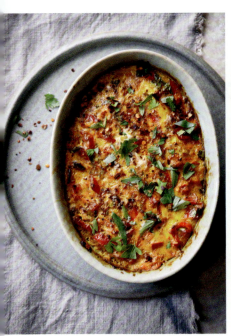

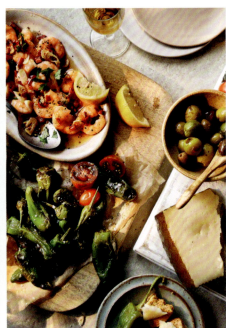

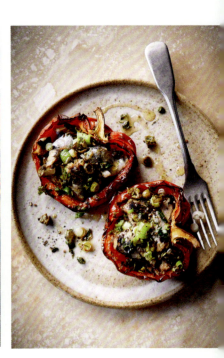

NIBBLES AND LIGHT MEALS

Spicy Nuts

Serves 4 (makes
120g/4¼oz)

According to studies, apparently eating just 20g (¾oz) of almonds
before a meal can reduce a blood glucose spike after a meal.
However, as they are high in fat and calories, and moreish, it can
be easy to overdo it. Measure out a portion and put them away
rather than leave them temptingly on the side. Serve them with
olives, celery or red pepper strips for a heartier snack.

1. Put the nuts into the drawer without a crisper or into a silicone
   liner or ovenproof dish in the drawer. Toss with the oil and all the
   flavourings until coated.

2. Air fry at 200°C (400°F) for 5–7 minutes until browned, tossing
   halfway through. Cool and store the nuts in a jar for up to a week.

120g (4¼oz) mixed nuts (such as
  almonds, hazelnuts, walnuts
  and pecans)
1 teaspoon extra-virgin olive oil
½ teaspoon salt
½ teaspoon Aleppo pepper or sweet
  smoked paprika
2 teaspoons finely chopped
  rosemary
¼ teaspoon chilli flakes or pinch
  of cayenne pepper

Per serving: 190kcal			
NET CARBS	FIBRE	PROTEIN	FAT
5g	2g	7g	16g

Cheesy Garlicky Kale Crisps

Use any firm green leaves from the cabbage family such as kale, cauliflower or even Brussels sprout leaves, which are often thrown away as waste. In a matter of minutes, the leaves become crisp. Don't wash the leaves unless they are muddy, in which case shake them well and dry them on kitchen paper. As a keen gardener, I have also used ground elder, nettles and basil leaves with great effect!

1. Roughly tear the kale leaves into bite-sized pieces – the same size as large potato crisps. Put these in a bowl with all the remaining ingredients and mix together using your hands or a large spoon. Spread them out over a crisper in the drawer (do this in batches if the drawer is small).

2. Air fry at 200°C (400°F) for 3 minutes. Toss, then cook again for 2–3 minutes until crisp.

3. Serve straight away or leave to cool. Any leftovers will keep for a couple of days in an airtight container. If they become soft, put them back into the air fryer for a couple of minutes to crisp up again.

200–250g (7–9oz) kale, ribs removed
1 teaspoon smoked paprika
¼ teaspoon salt
2 teaspoons black onion (nigella) seeds
1 teaspoon extra-virgin olive oil
1 teaspoon garlic granules
2 tablespoons finely grated Parmesan, Grana Padano or vegetarian Italian-style hard cheese
freshly ground black pepper

Tips and tricks
I have flavoured these with spices and cheese, but kale crisps are also great tossed with salt or a couple of teaspoons of tamari and olive oil.

For the flavour of crispy seaweed, use sesame oil instead of olive oil and add ½ teaspoon of ground ginger, ¼ teaspoon of chilli flakes and 1 teaspoon of sesame seeds, plus 2 teaspoons of soy sauce instead of the salt. Mix well with the kale and cook as above.

Per serving: 45kcal			
NET CARBS	FIBRE	PROTEIN	FAT
1g	3g	3g	3g

Halloumi Fries

Warm, gooey halloumi cheese is gorgeous. Serve these fries with Spicy Nuts, with red pepper or carrot sticks and Guacamole, or with Spicy Roasted Tomato Salsa or Avocado Cream (see pages 54, 194, 91 and 78). You can see from the protein and calories that this is more than snack food and should be consumed as part of a meal.

1. Preheat the air fryer with a crisper in the drawer to 200°C (400°F).

2. Mix the almonds with the paprika and onion seeds, if using, in a bowl.

3. Dry the halloumi chips with kitchen paper and then lay them on a plate. Spray them with oil, then turn and spray the other side. Dip the chips into the coating, making sure they are well covered.

4. Spray or brush the crisper with oil. Lay the chips on the prepared crisper and cook for 6–8 minutes. Serve straight away.

75g (2½oz) ground almonds
1 teaspoon smoked paprika
1 teaspoon black onion (nigella) seeds (optional)
250g (9oz) halloumi cheese, cut into even chips, cubes or slices
2 teaspoons extra-virgin olive oil

Per serving: 341kcal			
NET CARBS	FIBRE	PROTEIN	FAT
3g	1g	17g	29g

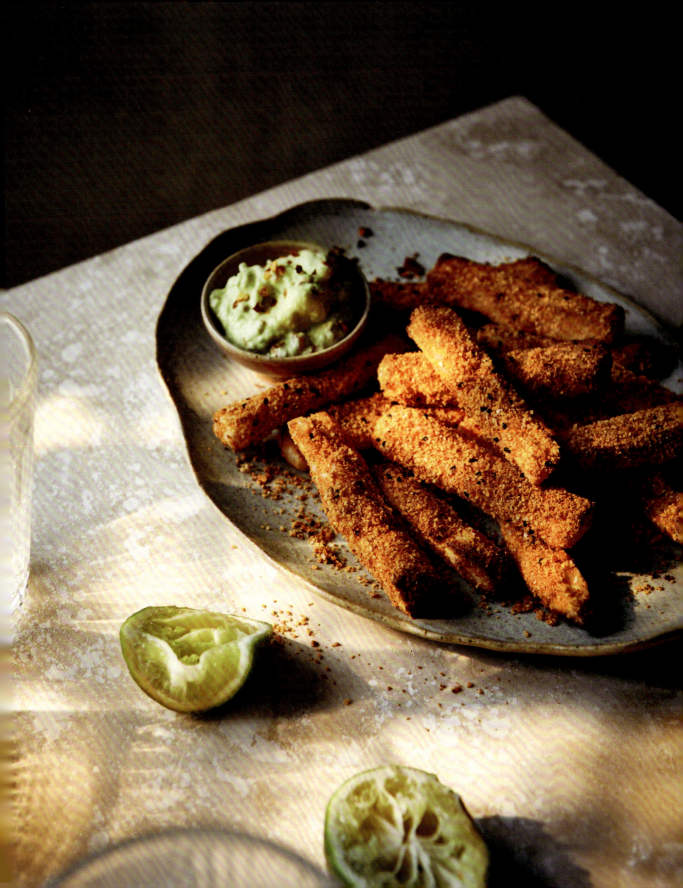

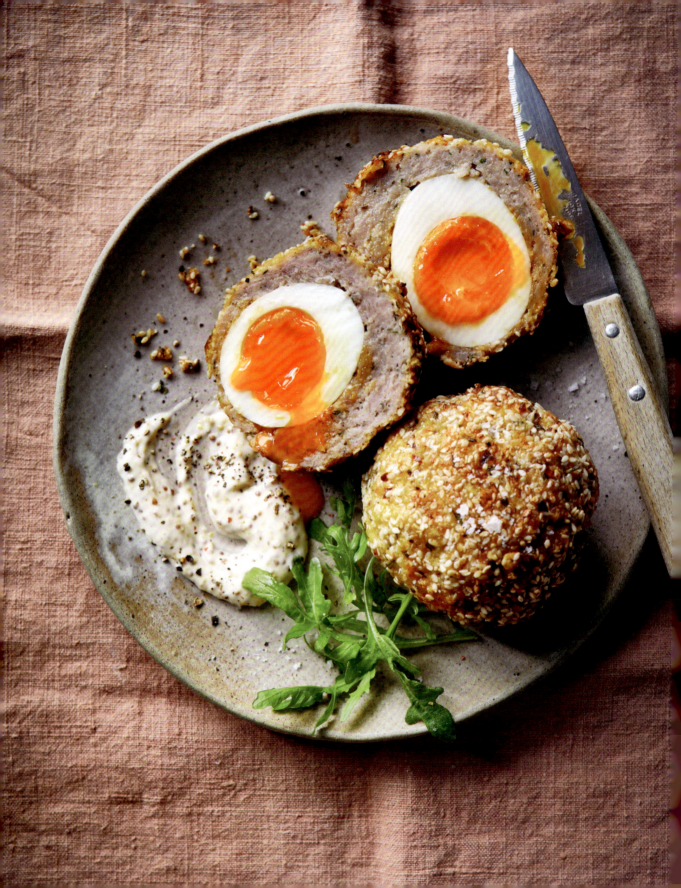

Scotch Eggs

Scotch eggs were invented by Fortnum and Mason in 1738 for travellers heading west from London on train journeys. Scotch eggs still make the perfect food to go today as they are robust and filling. I love to eat them with mustard, so I try to take this along with me, too. Add herbs if your sausagemeat doesn't already contain them.

1. Spray or brush a crisper in the drawer generously with oil. Score a line down the sausages, if using, and peel away the skins. Put the sausages or sausagemeat into a bowl and roughly divide into 4 portions.

2. To prepare the coating, mix all the dry ingredients together in another bowl. Crack and beat the egg in another bowl.

3. Take one portion of the sausagemeat and flatten it in your hand to just larger than your palm. Take a boiled egg and put it on the meat. Curl your hand around it and press it into a ball shape so that the egg is evenly covered with the meat. Repeat with the other portions of sausagemeat and boiled eggs. Wash and dry your hands.

4. Using one hand, dip each sausage-covered egg into the beaten egg to coat and then drop it into the dry mixture. Use the other hand to tip the bowl from side to side to coat the wet ball. Use the same dry hand to roll it around so that it is evenly coated. Lay the Scotch egg on a large plate and then repeat with the remaining sausage-covered eggs.

5. The Scotch eggs are best double-dipped to create a thicker, crisper coating, so take each one and repeat the process above, returning them to the plate.

6. Spray with oil from the top and put them, spaced apart, oil-side down, on the crisper. Spray the tops with oil.

7. Air fry at 200°C (400°F) for 7 minutes, or until richly golden brown. Turn the eggs and continue to cook for 5–7 minutes until richly golden brown all over.

8. Remove from the drawer and serve straight away or allow to cool to room temperature. Store in the refrigerator for up to 2 days.

extra-virgin olive oil
400g (14oz) high-meat-content sausages or sausagemeat
2 teaspoons finely chopped fresh or dried rosemary
60g (2¼oz) finely grated Parmesan, Grana Padano or Italian-style hard cheese
60g (2¼oz) sesame seeds
pinch of chilli flakes (optional)
1 egg
4 soft-boiled eggs, cooled and peeled (see page 43)

Per Scotch egg: 518kcal			
NET CARBS	FIBRE	PROTEIN	FAT
3g	2g	33g	42g

Berber-style Omelette

Traditionally, a Berber omelette is cooked in a tagine, the conical terracotta pot placed over a fire in Morocco. Inspired by her travels in Morocco, my friend Susanne brought this recipe home for me to try in an air fryer. It works brilliantly and, like most frittata/omelette/shakshuka-style eggs, can be altered to use up whatever you have in the refrigerator. I have added in chopped courgette or asparagus. To speed things up, use frozen, chopped garlic and ginger and vegetables straight from the freezer. Leave some or all of the eggs whole or break them up and stir them in, it's your omelette! This is often served with harissa on the side.

1. Place the shallot, pepper, chilli, oil and seasoning in a roughly 12–15cm (4½–6 inch) circular or oval ovenproof dish. Air fry at 200°C (400°F) for 7–10 minutes, depending on whether the vegetables are frozen or not.

2. Now add the tomatoes, garlic, ginger and ground spices, stirring them into the shallot mixture. Cook for a further 5–7 minutes until the tomatoes have collapsed and you have a rough, tomato sauce. Taste and add more seasoning accordingly.

3. Now stir in the chopped herbs, then crack the eggs into the sauce. Using a spatula, stir the whites around without breaking the yolks. Cook for a further 5 minutes, or until the eggs are done to your liking.

4. Lift the dish out with oven gloves, tongs or an angled slice and serve scattered with a few extra herbs.

1 shallot or 2 spring onions, finely chopped
1 Romano pepper or ½ red bell pepper, cored, deseeded and finely chopped, or 100g (3½oz) frozen chopped peppers
½–1 hot green chilli, according to strength, finely chopped
2 teaspoons extra-virgin olive oil
2 tomatoes, finely diced
1 garlic clove, grated, or 1 teaspoon frozen chopped garlic
2 teaspoons fresh or frozen grated root ginger
½ teaspoon ground cumin
¼ teaspoon ground turmeric
1 tablespoon chopped fresh coriander and/or parsley, plus extra to garnish
2 eggs
salt and pepper

Per serving: 316kcal			
NET CARBS	FIBRE	PROTEIN	FAT
18g	6g	15g	19g

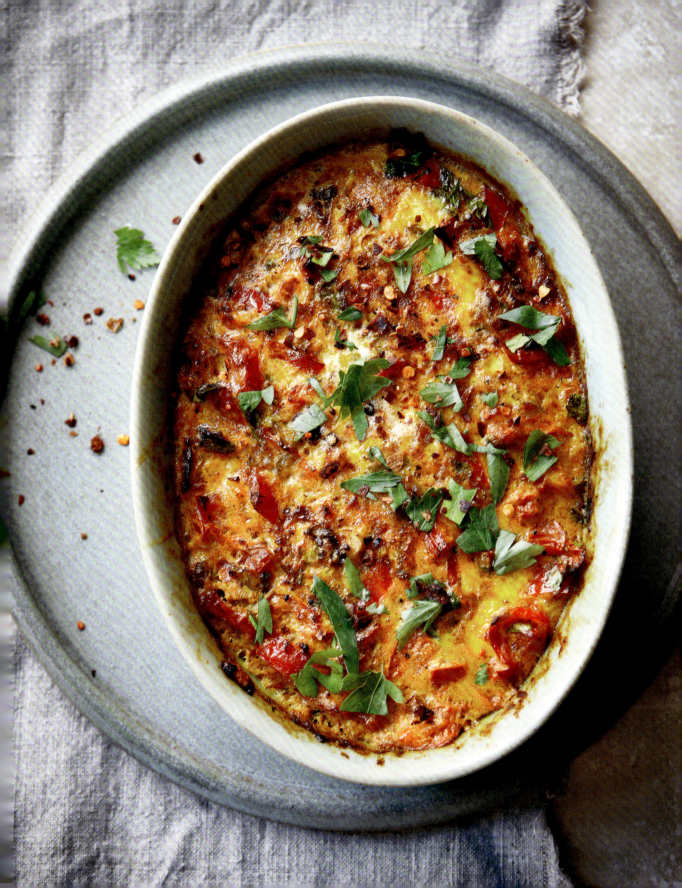

Quick Mushroom and Tahini Soup

Bowls of hot mushroom soup are perfect for chilly days, and air fryers make cooking mushrooms a doddle. With just a few sprays of oil, you can have tasty mushrooms in minutes. This soup is thickened by puréeing it with tahini rather than adding carby potatoes. I love the combo of tahini and mushrooms; like a perfect partnership, they enhance each other's qualities. Make it vegan with olive oil, vegetable stock and tofu, or use butter and cream and add chicken if you prefer (see below).

1. Preheat the air fryer to 200°C (400°F).

2. Put the butter in the drawer, then add the onion, celery, garlic, rosemary and a little salt and pepper. Air fry for 5–7 minutes, tossing twice in that time to coat the vegetables in the butter.

3. Add the mushrooms and stir through with a spatula. Return the drawer to the air fryer and cook for 8 minutes, or until the mushrooms are lightly browned and cooked.

4. Pour the hot stock and tahini into the drawer and stir through. If you like it smooth, transfer to a blender and whizz until smooth; or you can leave it rough and chunky. If using chicken (see below), stir it into the soup, return the drawer to the air fryer and cook for 5 minutes until piping hot. Taste the soup and add seasoning as necessary.

5. Serve the soup in bowls with a dollop of crème fraîche, yogurt, cream or tofu, if using, some chopped chives or parsley, if using, and a twist of pepper.

3 tablespoons butter or extra-virgin olive oil
1 small onion or leek, roughly chopped
1 celery stick, roughly chopped
2 garlic cloves, whole but lightly crushed
1 heaped teaspoon chopped fresh or dried rosemary or thyme
400g (14oz) chestnut or portobello mushrooms
600ml (20fl oz) hot vegetable stock
2 tablespoons tahini
salt and pepper

To serve
crème fraîche, Greek yogurt, double cream or blended silken tofu (optional)
a few chopped chives or parsley (optional)

Tips and tricks

For protein, you can add chicken, a couple of poached eggs or the Halloumi Croutons on page 104. The soup alone is low in protein, but these additional topping options add more:

50g (1¾oz) cooked and shredded chicken will give 15g protein and 0g net carbs.

2 medium eggs will give 11g protein and 1g net carbs.

1 serving of air-fried halloumi croutons will give 13g protein and 1g net carbs.

100g (3½oz) silken tofu will give 7g protein and 2g net carbs.

Per serving of soup for 4 without toppings: 159kcal			
NET CARBS	FIBRE	PROTEIN	FAT
6g	5g	2g	13g

Devilled Eggs

Serves 4

The punchy filling makes these traditional canapés a perfect low-carb recipe. Have as a light starter or make a meal of them with the Low-carb Bread on page 156.

1. Cut each egg in half and scoop out the yolks into a small bowl.

2. Mash the yolks with all the remaining ingredients using a fork until smooth. Taste and adjust the seasoning and heat as you like.

3. Spoon (or pipe) the mixture into the halved whites and serve scattered with cayenne pepper and a few more herbs.

4 hard-boiled eggs (see page 43), cooled and peeled
1 tablespoon mayonnaise, preferably homemade (see page 195)
1 tablespoon Greek yogurt
½ teaspoon white or red wine vinegar or a squeeze of lemon juice
1 teaspoon Dijon or English mustard
a few drops of Tabasco or other hot sauce
¼ teaspoon celery salt
1 tablespoon finely chopped chives or celery leaves, plus extra to serve
freshly ground black pepper
cayenne pepper, to serve

Per serving: 98kcal			
NET CARBS	**FIBRE**	**PROTEIN**	**FAT**
1g	0g	6g	8g

Curried Vegetable Soup with Crispy Paneer Croutons

This is such a quick and easy soup to make from a bag of frozen, chopped vegetables. I like the mix of green beans, carrots and sweetcorn, but any low-carb vegetables will do; just avoid too much sweet potato or butternut squash. Dried curry leaves can be used, but usually they lack flavour, so double the quantity. Fresh curry leaves are great to freeze, so buy them when you see them. To make this vegan, use olive oil for frying and tofu instead of the paneer. To make a thicker soup, use a stick blender to blitz one-third of it, adding hot water to obtain a good consistency.

1. Put the onion, garlic, ginger, chilli, ghee and some seasoning in the base of the drawer. Air fry at 180°C (350°F) for 5–7 minutes, or until softened, shaking the drawer halfway.

2. Add the curry powder and stir through before adding the frozen vegetables. Stir again and cook at 180°C (350°F) for 5 minutes, shaking the drawer halfway.

3. Now add the coconut milk, stock and curry leaves and cook at 160°C (325°F) for 35 minutes, or until the vegetables are tender. Taste the soup and add more spices or seasoning as necessary. If you only have 1 drawer, tip the soup into a saucepan to keep it warm while you fry the paneer just before serving.

4. Coat the paneer in olive oil and the onion seeds in a small bowl. Air fry at 200°C (400°F) for 5–8 minutes, or until golden brown and crisp, shaking the drawer a couple of times during the cooking time.

5. Serve the soup in bowls topped with the paneer cubes and coriander, if using. Once cooled, the soup will keep in the refrigerator for up to 3 days or in the freezer for up to 3 months.

1 onion, finely chopped
2 garlic cloves, finely chopped, or 2 teaspoons frozen garlic
15g (½oz) fresh root ginger, grated, or 1 tablespoon frozen ginger
1 hot green or red chilli, finely chopped, or 1 teaspoon chilli flakes
2 tablespoons ghee or 1 tablespoon butter plus 1 tablespoon olive oil
1 tablespoon curry powder (pick your favourite)
500g (1lb 2oz) mixed frozen vegetables
400g (14oz) can full-fat coconut milk
200ml (7fl oz) warm vegetable stock
10 fresh curry leaves
salt and pepper
fresh coriander leaves, to serve (optional)

For the crispy paneer croutons
200g (7oz) paneer, cut into 1.5cm (⅝ inch) cubes
extra-virgin olive oil
1 teaspoon black onion (nigella) seeds

	Per serving: 495kcal		
NET CARBS	FIBRE	PROTEIN	FAT
16g	6g	15g	38g

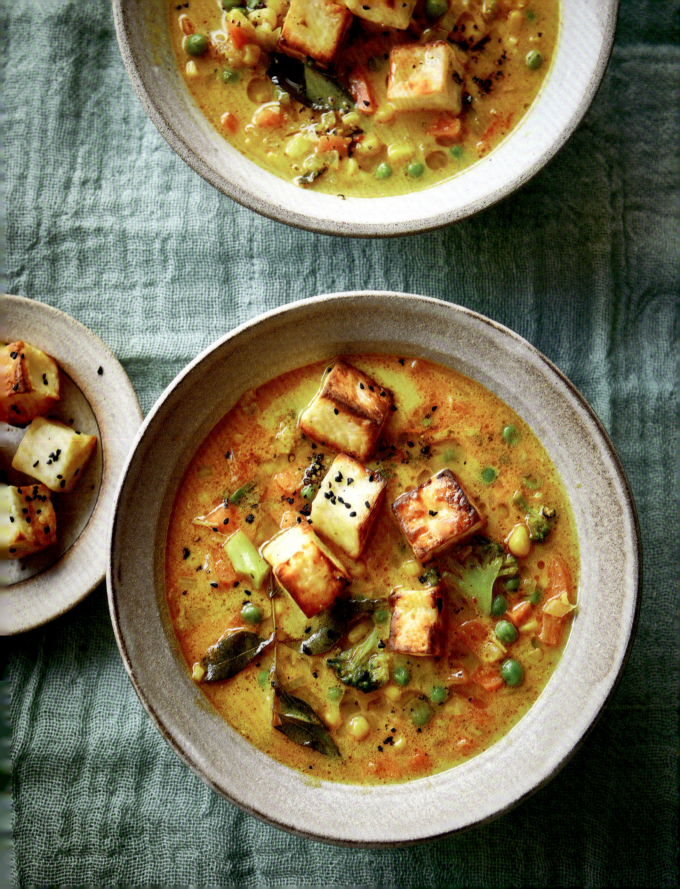

Tapas Platter (pictured overleaf)

We love a sharing platter when friends drop round, plus it gives me the excuse to buy more wooden chopping boards! If you are doing this in batches, keep the peppers or chorizo warm while you finish cooking. Cook the chorizo, peppers and mushrooms in the air fryer and add whatever you like inspired by Spanish holidays! Olives, Manchego cheese, Spicy Garlic and Parsley Prawns (see opposite).

Padrón Peppers

1. Scatter the peppers over a crisper, spray with the oil, then shake the drawer to coat the peppers with oil.

2. Put into the air fryer and cook at 200°C (400°F) for 5–7 minutes until the peppers are browned and lightly blistered, shaking once during cooking to turn them.

3. Tip the peppers on to a wooden board to serve with a bowl for the stalks. Scatter with salt flakes and serve.

130g (4½oz) Padrón peppers
1 teaspoon extra-virgin olive oil
salt flakes

Per serving: 7kcal			
NET CARBS	FIBRE	PROTEIN	FAT
0g	1g	1g	0g

Crispy Chorizo

1. Spread the chorizo on a crisper in one layer. Put into the air fryer and cook at 200°C (400°F) for 5–7 minutes until crisp.

2. Transfer the crispy slices with a slotted spoon to the serving board. Reserve the oil for the mushrooms.

300g (10½oz) cooking chorizo, cut into 5mm (¼ inch) slices (or use mini cooking chorizo sausages)

Per serving: 243kcal			
NET CARBS	FIBRE	PROTEIN	FAT
2g	0g	11g	21g

Spicy Mushrooms

This uses the deliciously flavoured oil left in the drawer from cooking the chorizo.

1. Remove the crisper and take a look at the oil left over from cooking the chorizo. You will need around 2 tablespoons, so if there isn't enough, make it up with olive oil, or use chilli oil if you are vegetarian. Toss the mushrooms in the oil, garlic and seasoning until evenly coated and then spread them out.

2. Put into the air fryer and cook at 200°C (400°F) for 7 minutes, or until cooked and lightly browned, tossing the mushrooms halfway through. Serve hot.

2 tablespoons leftover chorizo-flavoured oil (or use chilli oil)
250g (9oz) mushrooms, trimmed and sliced
1 garlic clove, grated
pinch of salt
freshly ground black pepper

Per serving: 73kcal			
NET CARBS	FIBRE	PROTEIN	FAT
1g	1g	2g	7g

Spicy Garlic and Parsley Prawns

Serves 2

(pictured overleaf)

This is a great quick dish to make with prawns straight from the freezer. Serve in bowls with a spoon to enjoy all the juices or have with the low-carb bread rolls on page 156.

1. Place the frozen prawns on a crisper in the drawer and air fry at 200°C (400°F) for 5 minutes to defrost. Use a spatula to transfer the prawns to a bowl. Remove the crisper and tip away the water. Fill a serving bowl with hot water to warm it.

2. Put the prawns, garlic, chilli, salt and butter or oil into the empty drawer without the crisper or into a silicone liner or ovenproof dish. Put it into the air fryer and cook at 200°C (400°F) for 2 minutes. Pull out the drawer and toss everything together to coat with the melted butter. Replace the drawer and cook for 2–4 minutes until the prawns are pink and cooked through.

3. Drain the warmed serving bowl, transfer the prawns to the bowl and stir in the parsley. Serve straight away with a squeeze of lemon.

250g (9oz) frozen raw peeled prawns
1 fat garlic clove, finely sliced
½–1 hot red or green chilli, finely chopped, or pinch of chilli flakes
¼ teaspoon salt
15g (½oz) butter or 1 tablespoon extra-virgin olive oil
small handful of parsley, stalks finely chopped and leaves roughly chopped
lemon wedges, to serve

Tips and tricks

Use whole prawns. If using frozen, defrost them first. Peel the shells off, leaving the heads intact, as this is where the flavour lies. Remove the black vein from the back of each one, then put the prawns and the rest of the ingredients into the empty drawer without a crisper or into a silicone liner or ovenproof dish and put into the air fryer at 200°C (400°F) for 2 minutes. Pull out the drawer and toss everything together with the melted butter or oil. Cook for 2–4 minutes until the prawns are pink and cooked through. Serve as above.

Per serving: 210kcal			
NET CARBS	**FIBRE**	**PROTEIN**	**FAT**
2g	0g	29g	9g

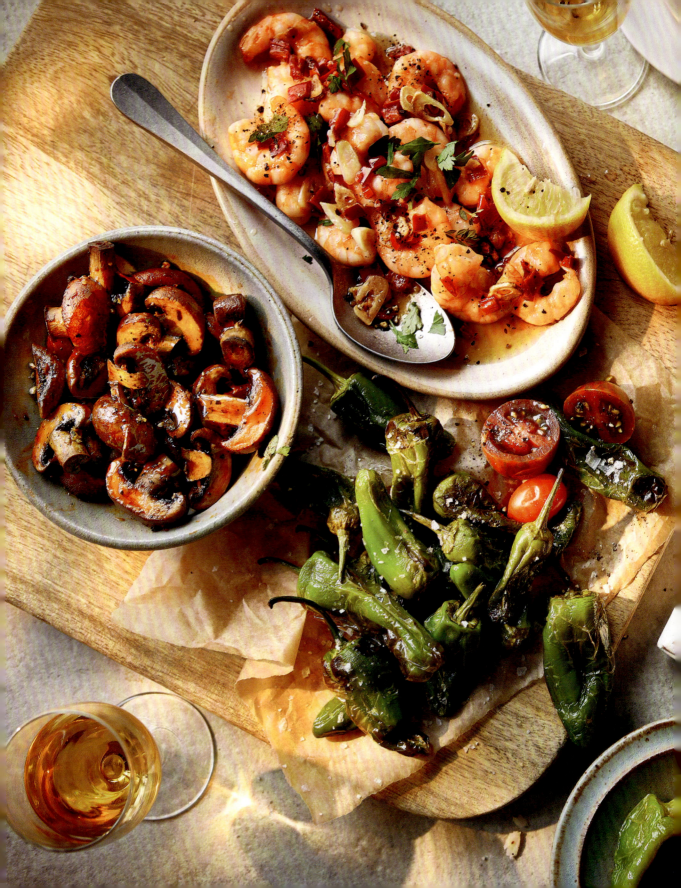

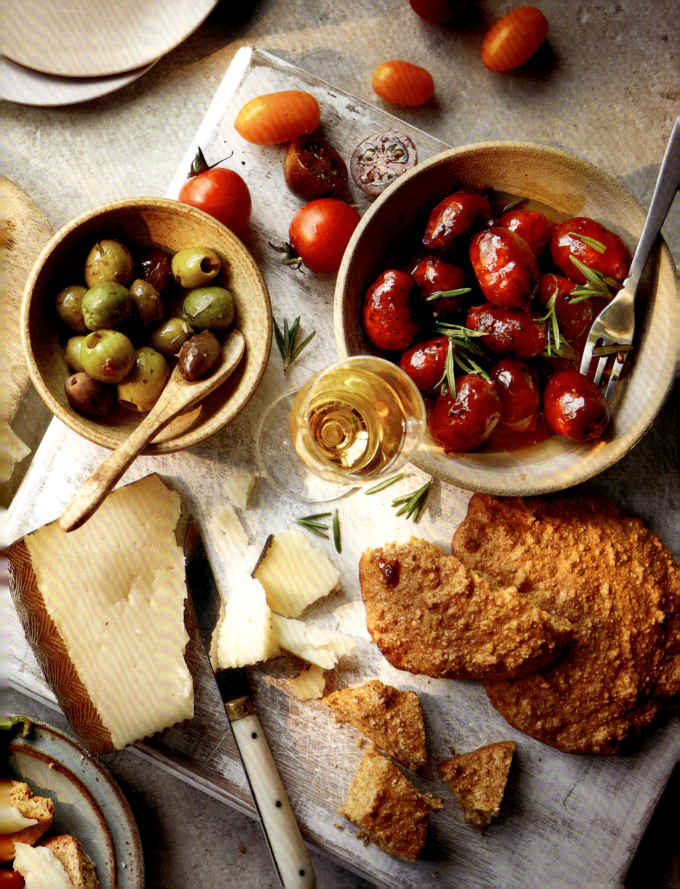

Charred Peppers on Cheat's Labneh

This stunning dish is good enough for a meal on its own or as part of a meal. It's great with the Low-carb Flatbreads on page 158. Labneh is a strained yogurt cheese available at some delis. If you can't find it easily, this makes an excellent substitute.

1. Put the peppers on a crisper in the drawer, brush with the oil and air fry at 200°C (400°F) for 30 minutes until blackened and blistered, turning once.

2. Put the peppers into a bowl and cover with a plate to sweat and cool.

3. Meanwhile, prepare the cheat's labneh by mashing the cheese and yogurt together in another bowl with a fork. Spread the labneh on to a plate and set aside.

4. Peel the skins from the peppers under water and discard along with the seeds and the cores. Tear the peppers into long strips and dry on a piece of kitchen paper. Lay them over the labneh, drizzle over the oil, season with salt and pepper and then scatter over the herbs. Chill in the refrigerator for up to an hour or serve straight away.

For the peppers
2 red peppers
2 teaspoons extra-virgin olive oil
salt and pepper

For the cheat's labneh
100g (3½oz) feta or goats' cheese
200g (7oz) thick Greek or strained
    yogurt
1 tablespoon extra-virgin olive oil
handful of fresh basil, coriander
    or flat leaf parsley leaves, or
    a mixture

Per serving: 196kcal			
NET CARBS	FIBRE	PROTEIN	FAT
6g	1g	7g	16g

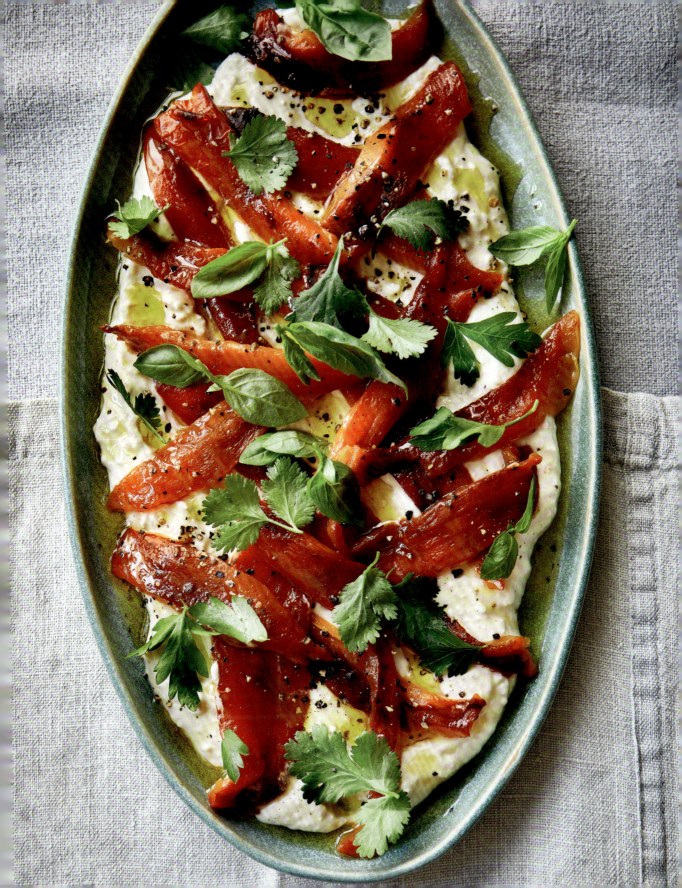

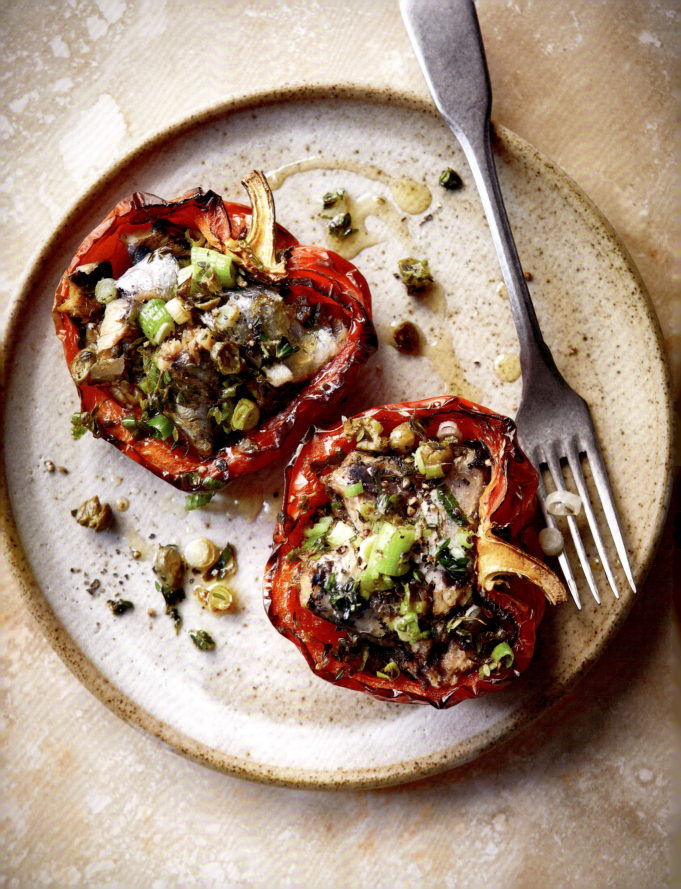

Sardines in Peppers

Deliciously quick sardines from the cupboard to your plate in minutes. While they cook, whip up a green salad with vinaigrette. Canned fish is overlooked but it is high in nutrition, especially protein and healthy fats, and it is low in cost.

1. Place the empty pepper shells, hollow-side up, on a crisper in the drawer and air fry at 200°C (400°F) for 8 minutes.

2. Meanwhile, mix 2 teaspoons of the oil in a bowl with some seasoning, the spring onion, oregano, capers and vinegar.

3. When the peppers are done, transfer them, hollow-side up, to an ovenproof dish (or 2) that will fit in your air fryer.

4. Put half the spring onion mixture into the shells, then top these with the sardines, dividing them between the peppers. Then add the last layer of spring onion mixture. Drizzle over the remaining teaspoon of the oil.

5. Air fry at 180°C (350°F) for 7–10 minutes until the pepper is soft and the sardines are hot. Serve straight away.

Tips and tricks
Add a pinch of chilli flakes if you like things spicy.

No sardines? Add canned mackerel fillets, tuna or salmon instead.

1 red pepper, halved lengthways, cored and deseeded
1 tablespoon extra-virgin olive oil
1 spring onion, finely chopped
1 teaspoon dried oregano or thyme
1 teaspoon capers, rinsed, chopped if large (optional)
1 teaspoon balsamic vinegar or red wine vinegar
1 can sardines (80g/2¾oz drained weight)
salt and pepper

Per serving: 231kcal			
NET CARBS	FIBRE	PROTEIN	FAT
5g	3g	22g	13g

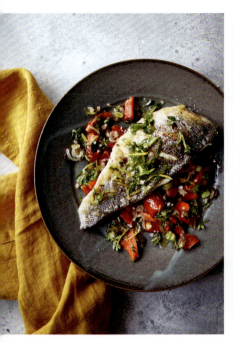
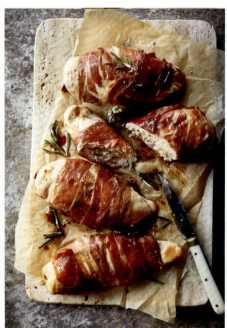
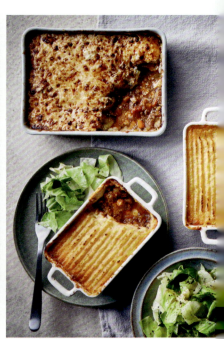

MAIN MEALS

Simple Fish Fillets

White fish fillets and oily fish, such as salmon, can be air fried but oily fish is less likely to dry out in the hot air passing around it. (See pages 81 and 86 for how to cook flat fillets such as seabass or seabream.) To cook vegetables with the fish, cut peppers into strips, broccoli into small florets or courgettes into slices, spray with oil and season, then lay them around the fish or under it using a rack.

1. Spray or brush a crisper in the drawer with oil.

2. Season the fish all over and add any flavourings, if using. Lay on the oiled crisper, then spray generously with oil. Air fry at 180°C (350°F) for 8–12 minutes, gently turning the fillet with a silicone spatula halfway through.

1 teaspoon extra-virgin olive oil
1 firm white fish (such as cod) or
    salmon fillet (approx. 120g/4¼oz)
flavourings (see below, optional)
salt and pepper

Tips and tricks

Cooking from frozen: Cook fillets at 180°C (350°F) for up to 15 minutes.

Spices: Add spices such as smoked paprika, ground cumin, chilli powder, baharat spice mix, Chinese 5 spice or curry powder.

A touch of umami: Drizzle the fish with tamari rather than using salt.

Rosemary and lemon butter: Mash 1 teaspoon of chopped fresh or dried rosemary, ½ teaspoon of finely grated lemon zest, a pinch of salt and some freshly ground black pepper into 10g (¼oz) of softened butter. Spread this on top of the fish halfway through cooking.

Per serving of cod: 176kcal			
NET CARBS	FIBRE	PROTEIN	FAT
0g	0g	30g	6g
Per serving of cod with rosemary and lemon butter: 248kcal			
NET CARBS	FIBRE	PROTEIN	FAT
0g	0g	30g	14g

Fish in a Parcel with Acqua Pazza Sauce

This classic Italian dish is served in a parcel to open at the table. Acqua Pazza means 'crazy water' as the sauce bubbles with heat and flavour. Cooking this way concentrates the flavours inside and prevents everything from becoming dry. It also means there is no washing up! This is best cooked with fresh or defrosted fish rather than frozen. Do two separate parcels or one large one depending on the size of your air fryer. If you can find them, buy capers in salt; they have a much better flavour than the ones in vinegary brine.

1. Cut 2 pieces of nonstick baking paper around 10cm (4 inches) bigger all around than your pieces of fish. Put the tomatoes, courgette, capers, herbs and chilli flakes into a bowl. Season cautiously with salt and pepper and toss through with a spoon to make sure the herbs are spread throughout.

2. Divide the tomato mixture between the 2 pieces of paper. Now season the fish all over and lay the fillets over the piles of tomatoes. Add the butter on top and bring the long edges of the paper together and fold them over by 2cm (¾ inch). Do this again and again until the paper fold sits around 5cm (2 inches) above the fish. Twist the ends like a sweet to trap in the steam and flavours.

3. Transfer to the drawer and air fry at 170°C (340°F) for 15 minutes, or until the fish feels firm to the touch through the paper.

4. Serve the fish on warm plates with the juices and parsley.

8 cherry tomatoes, quartered if large, halved if small
1 small courgette (approx. 200g/7oz), finely sliced
1 heaped tablespoon capers, rinsed
1 teaspoon dried oregano
1 teaspoon chopped fresh or dried thyme leaves
pinch of chilli flakes (optional)
280g (10oz) haddock, cod, whiting or other firm white fish or salmon fillets
2 tablespoons soft butter or extra-virgin olive oil
salt and pepper
a few parsley sprigs, roughly chopped, to serve

Per serving: 255kcal			
NET CARBS	FIBRE	PROTEIN	FAT
5g	3g	28g	14g

Giorgio's Spicy Salmon Cubes with Avocado Cream

Serves 2

Cool, creamy avocado or soured cream is great with this spicy, colourful salad bowl frequently cooked by our son Giorgio. Swap out the peppers for broccoli or cauliflower and the salmon for chicken breast or tofu (giving it a couple of minutes more if using chicken). The quick avocado cream can also be served as a dip or with drier dishes such as Falafel (see page 167) or fajitas (see page 90).

1. Mix the paprika together with the chilli powder or flakes, garlic, salt, plenty of pepper and the oil in a bowl. Add the salmon and vegetables and toss together. Put the salmon and veg on a crisper or into a silicone liner in the drawer and roast at 190°C (375°F) for 7 minutes, or until firm to the touch.

2. Meanwhile, make the avocado cream by halving and pitting the avocado and spooning out the flesh into a bowl. Using a fork, mash it with the yogurt, chilli and some salt and pepper. Squeeze the juice from one lime half into the cream and cut the other in half, so you have 2 wedges. Stir the cream, taste and add more salt or chilli as necessary.

3. Tip the salmon and vegetables into 2 bowls, add a spoonful of avocado cream, the lettuce, herbs, if using, and the lime wedges. Garnish with a sprinkle of chilli flakes.

1 teaspoon smoked paprika
pinch of chilli powder or flakes, plus extra to garnish
1 teaspoon fresh or frozen finely chopped garlic
¼ teaspoon salt
2 teaspoons extra-virgin olive oil
260g (9¼oz) salmon fillets, skinned and cut into 3cm (1¼ inch) cubes
2 spring onions, sliced, or 1 shallot, sliced into half moons
1 Romano pepper or ½ red bell pepper, cored, deseeded and cut into strips
freshly ground black pepper

For the avocado cream
1 ripe avocado
2 heaped tablespoons Greek yogurt
½ teaspoon chilli flakes, or freshly chopped chilli, or to taste
1 lime, halved
salt and pepper

To serve
1 little gem lettuce
handful of herbs, such as fresh coriander or parsley (optional)

Per serving of salmon: 331kcal			
NET CARBS	FIBRE	PROTEIN	FAT
3g	1g	34g	20g
Per serving of avocado cream: 143kcal			
NET CARBS	FIBRE	PROTEIN	FAT
4g	5g	3g	12g

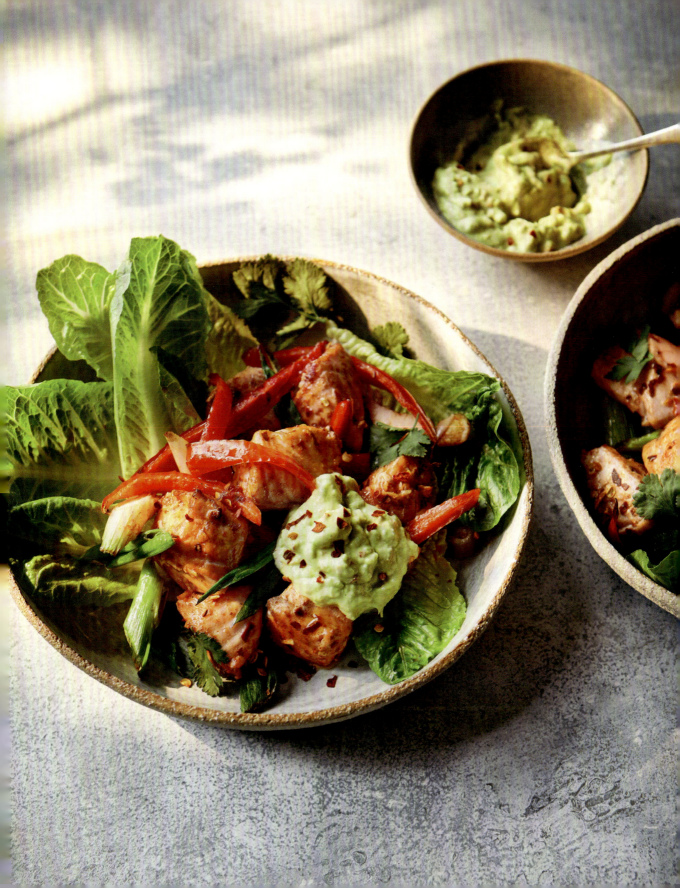

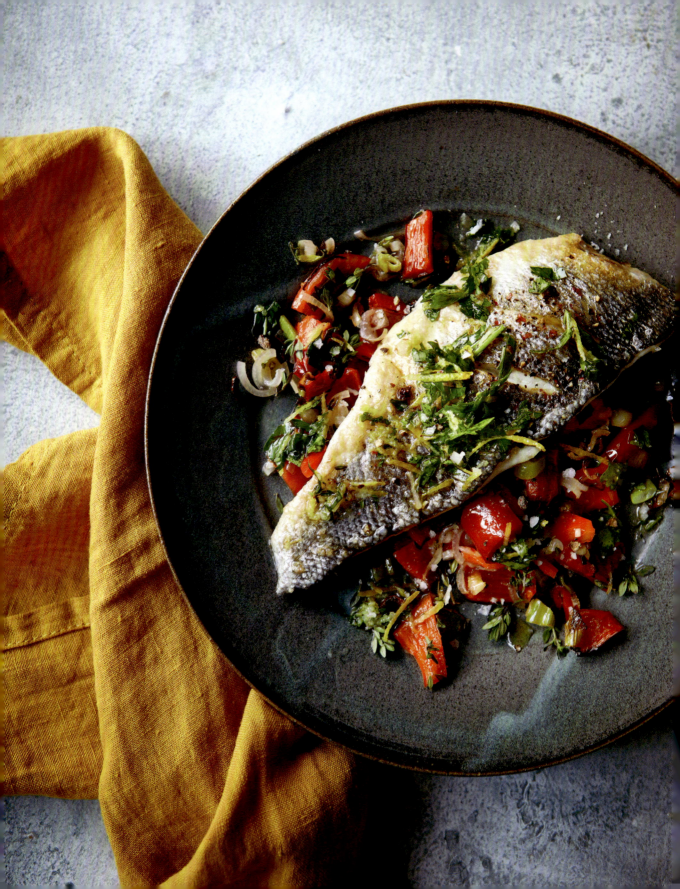

Seabass Fillets on Roasted Peppers with Lemon and Parsley Oil

Serves 2

This ridiculously simple supper can be made in 10 minutes; it is filling, delicious and looks pretty, too. The choice of herbs is up to you, but I can't resist a scattering here and there! Seabream or mackerel fillets also work great in this recipe. Any leftover lemon and parsley oil will keep in the refrigerator for up to 2 days.

1. Put the spring onions, garlic, thyme and half the oil in the drawer or in an ovenproof container with a little seasoning. Air fry at 200°C (400°F) for 2 minutes, or until just softened. Add the peppers and cook for a further 5 minutes. Toss the drawer to combine them with the oil and garlic once they have defrosted.

2. Place a rack or a crisper lightly over the peppers and put a piece of silicone or nonstick baking paper on top. Lay the fish fillets on a plate and spray or brush both sides generously with the remaining oil. Evenly scatter with salt and pepper. Place the fillets on the rack, skin-side up, and air fry at 200°C (400°F) for 8 minutes, or until firm to the touch. There is no need to turn them halfway through.

3. Meanwhile, make the lemon and parsley oil by mixing all the ingredients together in a small bowl, then adjust the seasoning and lemon to your liking. Alternatively, whizz it all together in a small food processor.

4. Remove the rack with an angled slice or the prongs of a fork and set aside over a plate. Divide the peppers between 2 warm plates. Use a silicone spatula or thin metal slice to transfer the fish to each plate, drizzle over a little lemon and parsley oil, then serve.

Tips and tricks
Frozen seabass: Flat fish defrost quickly and can be cooked from frozen, but be prepared to give them 2 minutes longer if not cooked all the way through.

3 spring onions, finely chopped, or 1 small onion, finely sliced
1 garlic clove, roughly chopped (optional)
1 thyme sprig or pinch of dried thyme (optional)
1 tablespoon extra-virgin olive oil
200g (7oz) frozen chopped red peppers or 1 red pepper, cored, deseeded and chopped
2 seabass or seabream fillets, skin on (90g/3¼oz each)
salt and pepper

For the lemon and parsley oil
small handful (approx. 3g/⅛oz) parsley, stalks and leaves finely chopped
1 teaspoon finely grated lemon zest, or more to taste
1 tablespoon lemon juice
2 tablespoons extra-virgin olive oil
salt and pepper

Per serving: 427kcal			
NET CARBS	FIBRE	PROTEIN	FAT
5g	2g	22g	35g

Main Meals

81

Fish with Tartare Sauce

The average portion of fish and chips can have up to 69g carbs. This version has just 10g. I have allowed time to make tartare sauce as I love the homemade version, but do skip this if you don't have the ingredients. Serve with celeriac fries (see page 141) – if you have a dual drawer air fryer, make these while the fish cooks.

1. Spray or brush a crisper in the drawer with a little of the oil. Preheat the air fryer to 200°C (400°F).

2. Mix the almonds with the paprika, salt and some pepper in a bowl. Tip the mixture on to a plate and spread out. Break the egg into a shallow bowl and beat with a fork.

3. If the fish isn't already portioned, cut into 2 pieces and evenly season with a little salt. Dip into the beaten egg, followed by the almond mixture to coat. Lay the fish on a plate and spray oil on top.

4. Put the fish pieces, oiled-side down, on the crisper and spray the tops with oil. Air fry for 10–12 minutes, or until the fish feels firm to the touch.

5. While the fish is cooking, make the tartare sauce by mixing all the ingredients together in a bowl and adding the lemon juice to taste.

6. Top the tartare sauce with some chopped parsley, if liked, then serve the fish and sauce with the celeriac fries and lemon wedges.

1 teaspoon extra-virgin olive oil
50g (1¾oz) ground almonds
2 teaspoons mild paprika
½ teaspoon salt, plus extra to serve
1 egg
240g (8½oz) haddock, cod or other firm white fish fillets, skinned
freshly ground black pepper

For the tartare sauce
2 tablespoons shop-bought or homemade mayonnaise (see page 195)
1 tablespoon capers, rinsed, drained and roughly chopped
1 gherkin (finger size), roughly chopped
1 teaspoon lemon juice, or to taste
chopped parsley, to garnish (optional)

To serve
celeriac fries (see page 141)
lemon wedges

Per serving of fish: 317kcal			
NET CARBS	FIBRE	PROTEIN	FAT
3g	3g	30g	20g
Per serving of celeriac fries: 115kcal			
NET CARBS	FIBRE	PROTEIN	FAT
7g	3g	2g	3g
Per serving of tartare sauce: 103kcal			
NET CARBS	FIBRE	PROTEIN	FAT
0g	0g	0g	11g

The Diabetes Air Fryer Cookbook

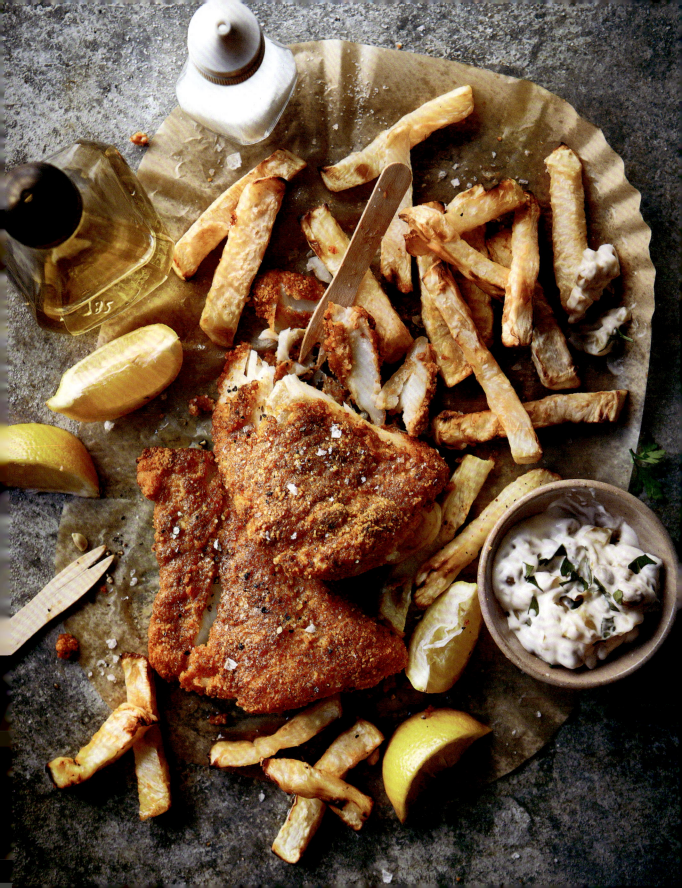

Teriyaki-style Salmon Stir Fry

Serves 2

Tasked with the job of preparing low-sugar foods for her family, our friend Debi put her twist on this delicious sauce for salmon, firm tofu or chicken. Use any vegetables you have in the refrigerator, replace the salmon with chicken or tofu, toss and serve in bowls. Debi's twist is to add Shaoxing rice wine instead of mirin, as it is sugary, and mustard to thicken the sauce. Konjac noodles are made from a root. They have been used in Japan for years and have zero carbs and calories. They are available in most supermarkets and are sometimes called 'zero', 'slim', 'diet' or 'skinny' noodles. Swap the salmon for the same weight of tofu or chicken if preferred.

1. To make the teriyaki sauce, combine all the ingredients with 2 tablespoons water in a small saucepan. Bring to the boil, then reduce the heat and simmer for 5 minutes. Remove from the heat, pour into a mixing bowl and leave to cool.

2. When the teriyaki sauce is at room temperature, stir the salmon through it. Cover and put it into the refrigerator to marinate for 10–30 minutes.

3. In a bowl, toss all the vegetables in the oil with salt and pepper.

4. Line the drawer with nonstick baking paper or with a silicone liner. Put the salmon into it and air fry at 200°C (400°F) for 8 minutes, or until lightly browned and firm to the touch. Cook the vegetables in a lined drawer at 200°C (400°F) for 6–8 minutes, or until tender, stirring halfway through.

5. Bring a pan of water to the boil. Put the rinsed konjac noodles into the pan and boil for 2 minutes, then drain.

6. Gently toss the salmon, vegetables and noodles in bowls. Serve scattered with sesame seeds, if using.

For the teriyaki sauce
1 tablespoon dark soy sauce
1 teaspoon honey or 2 teaspoons erythritol
1 teaspoon grated or finely chopped fresh root ginger
1 teaspoon grated or finely chopped garlic
½ red chilli, chopped, or pinch of chilli flakes
1 teaspoon sesame oil
2 teaspoons Shaoxing rice wine or dry sherry
½ teaspoon Dijon mustard
salt and pepper

For the stir fry
350g (12oz) salmon fillets
½ red pepper, cored, deseeded and roughly diced
100g (3½oz) green vegetables (such as asparagus, courgette or broccoli), cut into bite-sized pieces
2 spring onions, roughly diced
2 teaspoons sesame or extra-virgin olive oil
250g (9oz) konjac noodles, rinsed
salt and pepper
1 teaspoon black or white sesame seeds, toasted, to serve (optional)

Per serving with salmon: 505kcal			
NET CARBS	FIBRE	PROTEIN	FAT
10g	6g	47g	29g

Tuna and Mozzarella Burgers

For this recipe, I use blocks of firm, inexpensive cows' milk mozzarella, which grates easily. If you have only the soft type, it will also work but is slightly fiddlier to grate. Freeze any remaining mozzarella. Don't worry if your can of tuna provides up to 150g (5½oz) of tuna once drained; it will be fine. Keep these plain or add the chilli to flavour them as you wish. These patties set firm once cooled, so can be stored cooked in the refrigerator for up to 3 days, or frozen for up to 3 months. Use the spare egg white for the Granola on page 34 or the Mini Hazelnut and Chocolate Bites on page 182, or freeze it.

1. Oil a silicone paper liner or a piece of nonstick baking paper (cut to the size of the crisper so that the edges don't flap around).

2. Coarsely grate the mozzarella into a bowl; it will be messy if you are using the soft version but don't worry about that. Add the drained tuna, the spring onion, chilli, if using, egg yolk and seasoning. Use a fork to mash the ingredients together.

3. Roughly divide the mixture into 2 and use your hands to form each half into a ball, then flatten it out firmly, squeezing out any juice. Neaten them into patties measuring no more than 2cm (¾ inch) thick and lay on the oiled liner or paper.

4. Air fry at 200°C (400°F) for 8 minutes, or until lightly browned and firm to the touch. Use a silicone spatula to carefully flip the burgers over to the other side and cook for another 4 minutes, or until lightly browned. Leave the burgers to sit for 5 minutes to firm up before removing from the drawer.

5. Serve warm with salad.

Tips and tricks

Add 1 teaspoon of ground cumin or curry powder to the mixture. Alternatively, add 1 tablespoon of finely chopped herbs, such as fresh coriander or parsley.

extra-virgin olive oil, for greasing
100g (3½oz) firm mozzarella cheese
110g (3¾oz) drained tuna in brine
1 spring onion (approx. 10g/¼oz), finely chopped
¼–½ green chilli, finely chopped, or pinch of chilli flakes (optional)
1 egg yolk
salt and pepper

Per burger: 207kcal			
NET CARBS	FIBRE	PROTEIN	FAT
1g	0g	25g	11g

Bob's Curried Basa Fillets

Our friend Surinder (aka Bob) loves to make quick and easy Indian-style dishes. This quick fix for a weeknight supper is delicious. It uses inexpensive white fish fillets that can be bought in most supermarkets and Greek yogurt, which is high in protein and low in carbs. Serve it with a simple salad, such as Turkish Chopped Salad or Cucumber Raita, or with Cauliflower Rice (see pages 202, 195 and 199).

1. Mix the onion with 2 teaspoons of the olive oil in a bowl and a pinch of salt until coated. Transfer into the bottom of the air fryer drawer. Cook at 200°C (400°F) for 5 minutes.

2. In the same bowl, mix the yogurt with the spices, tomato purée, garlic and salt. Taste and adjust the flavour according to your taste, by adding more curry powder, chilli and/or salt as necessary.

3. Place a rack over the onion. Now put the fish fillets on a plate and coat one side with the yogurt mixture using a spoon. Spread the yogurt evenly over the fish and repeat on the other side so both fillets are covered.

4. Spray or drizzle the top of the fish with the remaining teaspoon of olive oil and place the fillets on the rack above the onion. Air fry the fish at 200°C (400°F) for 10 minutes. By this time, the fish should have just started to brown and the onion softened. If not, turn the air fryer up to 240°C (475°F) or as high as it will go and give it another 2 minutes to achieve a tandoori-baked appearance.

5. Serve warm with lemon wedges.

1 onion, finely sliced
1 tablespoon extra-virgin olive oil
30g (1oz) full-fat Greek yogurt
2 teaspoons your favourite curry powder, or more to taste
⅛–¼ teaspoon chilli powder or chilli flakes, or more to taste
1 tablespoon tomato purée
1 fat garlic clove, grated or finely chopped
2 skinless basa, tilapia, seabass or seabream fillets (250g/9oz total weight)
salt
lemon wedges, to serve

Per serving: 172kcal			
NET CARBS	FIBRE	PROTEIN	FAT
6g	1g	15g	10g

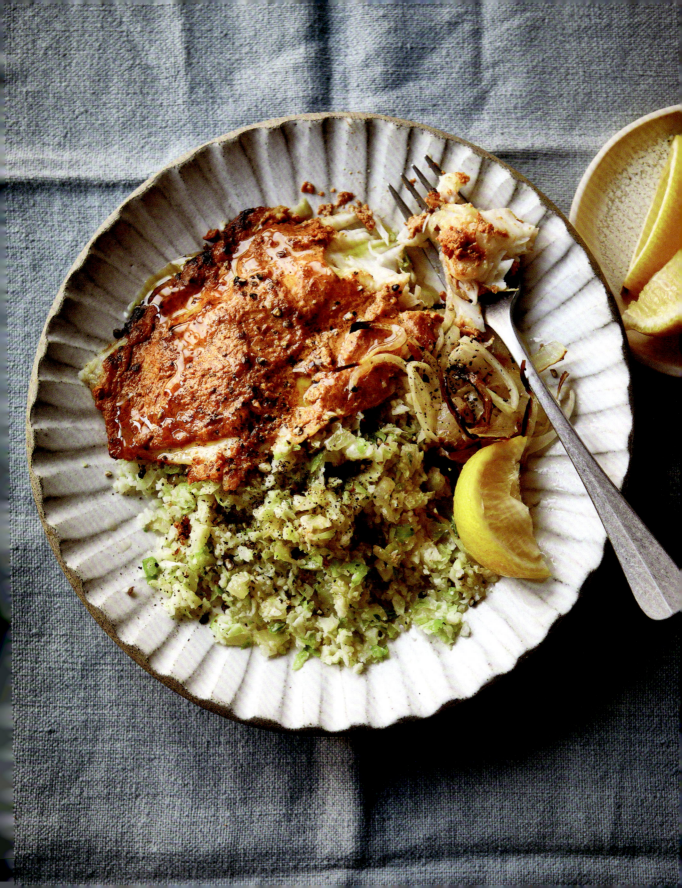

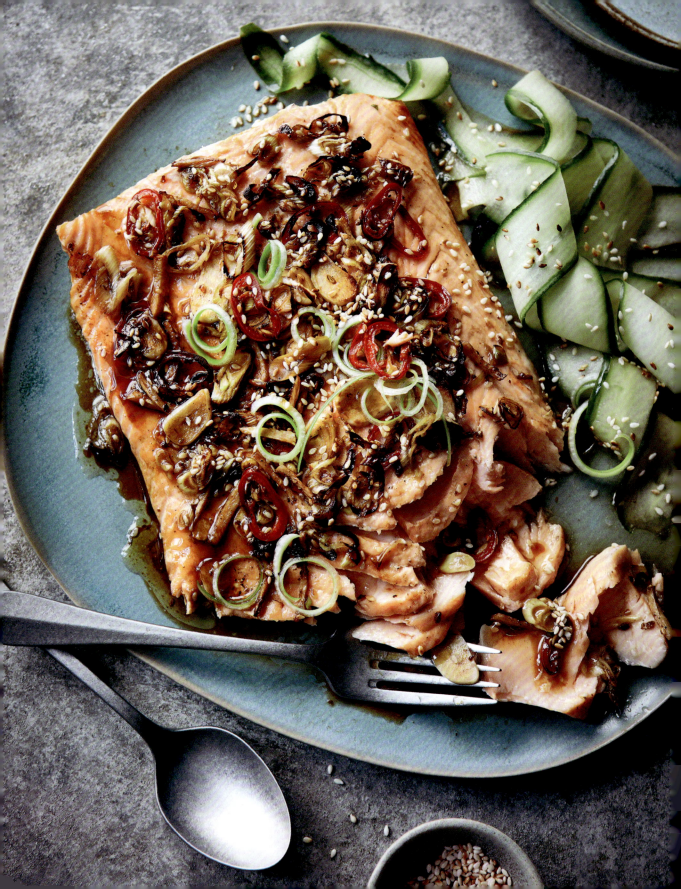

Roast Salmon with Ginger, Lemon Grass and Spring Onions

Serves 4

This stunning salmon dish is easy to make, and the spring onions and topping can be prepared in advance. Serve with cucumber ribbons made with a vegetable peeler, Cauliflower Rice (see page 199) or a green salad. I cheat with ready-chopped frozen ginger and garlic to make this dish even easier to prepare.

1. For the garnish, cut the green parts off the spring onions and slice lengthways through them but keeping one end intact. Put into cold water in a bowl to soak and curl while you prepare the rest.

2. Cut the remaining white parts diagonally and put them into a bowl with the lemon grass, sesame oil, tamari, pepper, chilli, ginger, garlic and sesame seeds. Stir through and set aside.

3. Put the salmon (if using fillets, push them together) on a baking paper liner in the drawer. Spray or brush with the olive oil. Roast at 180°C (350°F) for 10 minutes, or until firm to the touch and just cooked through.

4. Stir the ingredients in the bowl and tip these over the salmon. Air fry at 200°C (400°F) for 5 minutes, or until lightly browned and softened.

5. Transfer the salmon (leaving it in the paper, if you like) to a warm serving dish. Drain the green spring onion curls, pull them apart and scatter over the salmon. Garnish with sesame seeds, then serve.

4 spring onions
1 lemon grass stick, finely sliced
1 teaspoon toasted sesame oil
1 tablespoon tamari or dark soy sauce
1 teaspoon Szechuan pepper, crushed, or freshly ground black pepper
½–1 hot red chilli, finely sliced on the diagonal, or pinch of chilli flakes
10g (¼oz) fresh root ginger, peeled and cut into matchsticks, or 2 teaspoons frozen chopped ginger
1 fat garlic clove, finely sliced, or 2 teaspoons frozen chopped garlic
1 tablespoon sesame seeds, plus extra to garnish
600g (1lb 5oz) salmon, in one piece or fillets
2 teaspoons extra-virgin olive oil

Per serving: 367kcal			
NET CARBS	FIBRE	PROTEIN	FAT
2g	1g	39g	22g

Chicken Fajitas and Spicy Roasted Tomato Salsa in Lettuce Wraps

Serves 4

Make this dish as easy or as complex as you wish. For a quick supper for two, make half the recipe and enjoy the chicken, pepper and onion wrapped in lettuce leaves. For friends, go the whole way and make some or all of the following: Guacamole on page 194, or the Avocado Cream on page 78, the Spicy Roasted Tomato Salsa opposite, a jar of jalapeños, grated cheese, soured cream and fresh coriander.

Fajita seasoning often contains both chilli powder and cayenne pepper; both are hot, so if you choose to use both, add to taste. For a vegan alternative, use 500g (1lb 2oz) firm tofu instead of the chicken and leave out the soured cream and the cheese.

1. Prepare the marinade by combining all the spices with the oregano, salt, oil and garlic in a large mixing bowl. Add the chicken, red pepper and onion and toss well to coat everything. You can either cook this straight away or leave the flavours to meld together for up to an hour in the refrigerator.

2. Line 1 or 2 drawers, depending on the capacity of your air fryer, with baking paper liners. Air fry the mixture, sprayed with the oil, at 200°C (400°F) for 10 minutes, or until the chicken is cooked through. Check the chicken is done by cutting the thickest piece in half and making sure there are no pink juices running from it.

3. Serve the chicken, guacamole, tomato salsa, grated cheese, pickled jalapeños, soured cream and coriander sprigs in bowls on a large wooden board or on the table with the lettuce. Roll up a little of everything in a lettuce leaf and enjoy.

For the marinade
½ teaspoon chilli powder and/or cayenne pepper
1 teaspoon smoked paprika
1 teaspoon ground cumin
1 teaspoon dried oregano
1 teaspoon salt
1 tablespoon extra-virgin olive oil
1 garlic clove, grated, or 1 teaspoon garlic granules

For the fajitas
500g (1lb 2oz) boneless, skinless chicken breasts or tenders, cut into 2cm- (¾ inch)-long strips
1 red pepper, cored, deseeded and cut into strips
1 red onion, sliced
1 tablespoon extra-virgin olive oil

To serve
Guacamole (see page 194)
⅔ quantity of Spicy Roasted Tomato Salsa (see opposite)
50g (1¾oz) Cheddar or feta cheese, coarsely grated
pickled sliced jalapeños
50g (1¾oz) soured cream
small handful of fresh coriander sprigs
1 head of romaine or iceberg lettuce, trimmed and separated into leaves

Per serving of fajitas: 229kcal			
NET CARBS	FIBRE	PROTEIN	FAT
3g	1g	30g	10g
Per serving of soured cream: 25kcal			
NET CARBS	FIBRE	PROTEIN	FAT
1g	0g	0g	2.4g
Per serving of Cheddar: 75kcal			
NET CARBS	FIBRE	PROTEIN	FAT
1g	0g	3g	7g

Spicy Roasted Tomato Salsa

Air fryers are brilliant for quickly roasting vegetables. This spicy cooked salsa, or *salsa roja* in Spanish, will keep in the refrigerator for up to 3 days, so I always make a little more than needed; it's the perfect partner for fish, steak, Halloumi Fries (see page 56) or the fajitas opposite. There is no added sugar in this recipe, unlike in many shop-bought varieties. Use any tomatoes you have; it's a good way to use up those that are just going soft. If you don't like coriander, use parsley or basil leaves instead.

1 teaspoon olive oil
1 small onion, cut into 8 wedges
1 fat garlic clove, unpeeled and lightly crushed with the flat of a knife
300g (10½oz) tomatoes, halved
1 fresh jalapeño or hot red or green chilli, or more to taste, roughly chopped
¼ teaspoon ground cumin
juice of ½ lime
10g (¼oz) fresh coriander, leaves and stalks
¼–½ teaspoon salt, or more to taste

1. Spray or brush a crisper in the drawer with oil. Put the onion, garlic and tomatoes on the crisper and spray with oil. Roast at 200°C (400°F) for 15 minutes, or until starting to brown and are softened, moving the vegetables around halfway through and removing the garlic if it starts to burn.

2. Peel the garlic while the vegetables cool for 10 minutes, then transfer them to a blender with the remaining ingredients. Whizz to form a rough salsa. Taste and adjust more heat or salt as necessary.

Per serving: 24kcal			
NET CARBS	FIBRE	PROTEIN	FAT
3g	1g	1g	1g

Ham-wrapped Chicken Breasts with Cheese and Spring Onions

This restaurant-standard dish is easy to make but looks impressive. It's great for date nights or dinner parties (just double the recipe to serve 4). Look for inexpensive cream cheese that contains pure milk rather than emulsifiers and stabilizers. Use up the rest on any of the bread recipes (see pages 156–162) or on the Savoury Feta and Black Onion Seed Muffins on page 171. The ham or bacon adds fat to the chicken breasts, ensuring it doesn't dry out during cooking. If you don't want to use it, loosely wrap the chicken breasts in tin foil while cooking. This goes well with vegetables such as Creamy Spinach with Nutmeg or Asparagus, Tomatoes and Lemon (see pages 151 and 145).

1. Spray or brush the crisper with oil.

2. Make the stuffing by mixing the cream cheese with the spring onions and herbs and lemon zest, if using.

3. To stuff the chicken breasts, cut a 'pocket' around 5–6cm (2–2½ inches) wide along the length of each breast on the thinner edge, being careful not to cut all the way through. Open up the pocket and spoon half the filling into each breast. Close the pocket and wrap each breast with the ham or bacon rashers to keep the filling inside.

4. Place the chicken breasts in the prepared drawer. Spray or brush them both generously with oil and then roast them at 180°C (350°F) for 18 minutes, or until the internal temperature measures 75°C (167°F) (or check they are done by piercing the thickest part with a skewer and making sure there are no pink juices running from it).

5. Let the chicken breasts rest for 5 minutes, then serve with vegetables along with the juices from the drawer.

extra-virgin olive oil
50g (1¾oz) cream cheese
2 spring onions, finely chopped
1 teaspoon finely chopped thyme
   or rosemary leaves (optional)
1 teaspoon finely grated lemon zest
   (optional)
2 boneless, skinless chicken breasts
   (approx. 300g/10½oz)
4 slices of Parma or Serrano ham
   or 8 streaky bacon rashers
salt and pepper

Per serving: 367kcal			
NET CARBS	FIBRE	PROTEIN	FAT
3g	0g	45g	18g

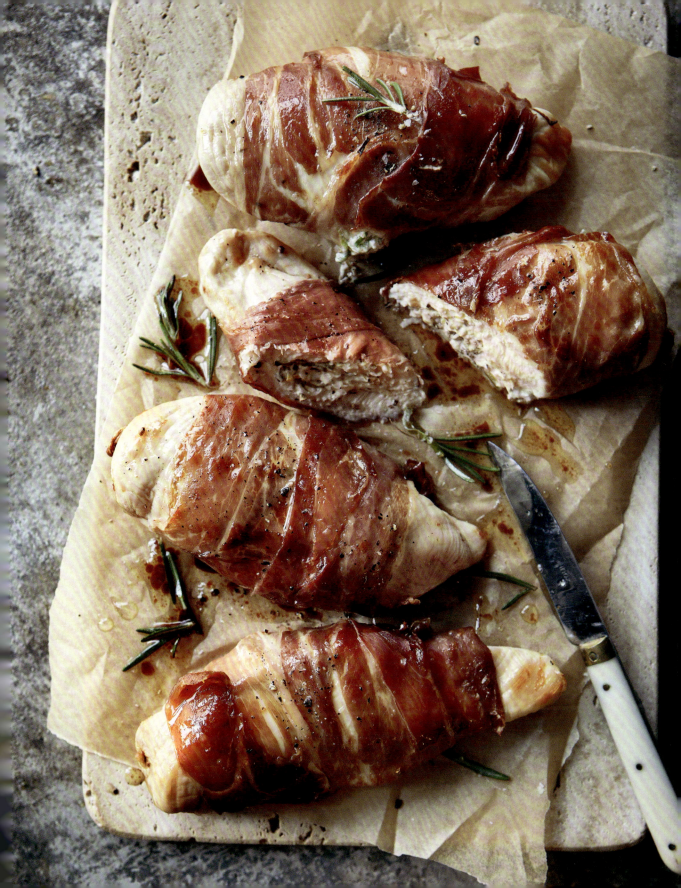

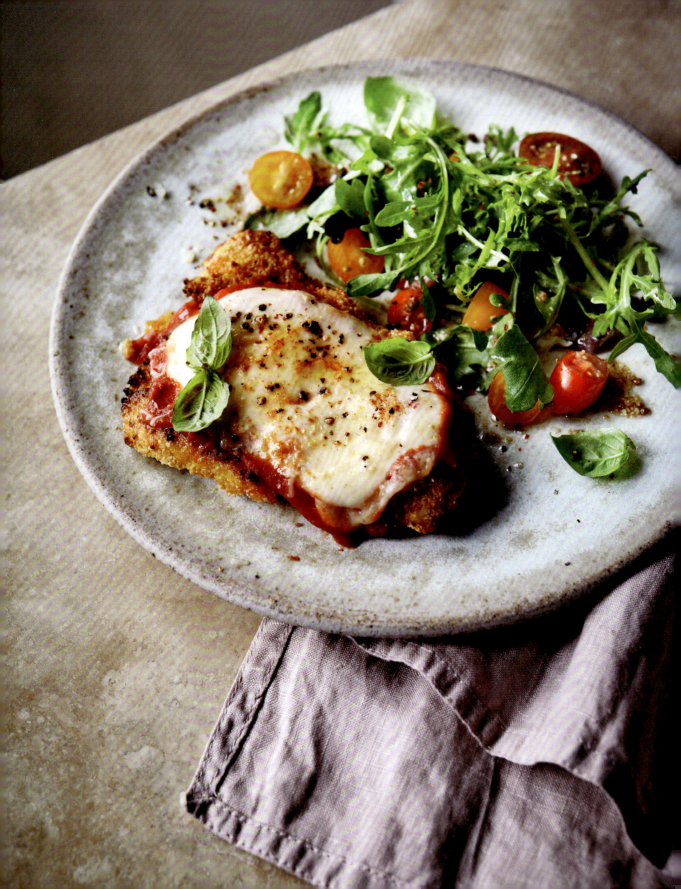

Chicken Parmigiana

This American-Sicilian classic dish was originally made with aubergines, while those who could afford it used meat. The aubergine recipe made its way to America with the Italians who emigrated there after the Second World War, and then as they prospered, it was replaced with chicken or veal. Usually it is made with breadcrumbs but I have swapped them for ground almonds. All this needs is a simple salad or green vegetables to go with it.

1. Cut the chicken breasts in half lengthways along the sides and open them up like a book. Cut through the spine of each 'book' so that you have 2 separate halves. Place the halves between 2 pieces of nonstick baking paper and pound the chicken breasts with a meat tenderizer or the base of a small saucepan until they are around 5mm (¼ inch) thick. Season evenly with salt and pepper and scatter half the oregano over the flattened chicken, pressing it in with your hands. Turn the chicken breasts over and season the other side, then scatter with the other half of the oregano.

2. Fold a piece of tin foil in two, long enough to push into the drawer under the crisper and out the other side to form a sling, to help lift out the hot crisper and chicken later. Lay this into the drawer and put a crisper on top. The ends of the tin foil should stick up around 4cm (1½ inches) above the crisper. Spray or brush the crisper with oil.

3. Prepare 3 wide bowls: one with the flour, one with the beaten eggs and one with the almonds mixed with half the Parmesan. Dip the chicken breast pieces first in the flour, shaking off any excess, then in the egg and then in the almond mixture, making sure they are evenly coated. Lay the chicken pieces on the crisper and spray with oil. Air fry at 200°C (400°F) for 10 minutes, or until cooked through. Pierce the chicken at the thickest part with a skewer and if there are any pink juices, cook for another 5 minutes. Alternatively, use a temperature probe to ensure the chicken is at least 75°C (167°F) inside the thickest part.

4. Spoon a heaped tablespoon of tomato sauce over each piece of chicken. Arrange the mozzarella on top of the chicken, scatter over the remaining Parmesan and some peper and bake at 200°C (400°F) for 4 minutes, or until the cheese is melted and the chicken is cooked through (check it is done by piercing the thickest part with a skewer and making sure there are no pink juices running from it). Carefully remove from the drawer using the tin foil sling and serve straight away topped with the basil leaves and some dried oregano.

400g (1lb 5oz) boneless, skinless chicken breasts
2 teaspoons dried oregano, plus extra to sprinkle
2 teaspoons extra-virgin olive oil
35g (1¼oz) chickpea flour
2 eggs, beaten
75g (2½oz) ground almonds
40g (1½oz) finely grated Parmesan, Grana Padano or Italian-style hard cheese
75g (2½oz) Classic or Roast Tomato Sauce (see pages 196 and 124) or passata (sieved tomatoes)
75g (2½oz) mozzarella cheese, cut into 1cm (½ inch) slices and drained in a sieve
salt and pepper
a few basil leaves, to garnish

Per serving: 491kcal			
NET CARBS	FIBRE	PROTEIN	FAT
9g	3g	46g	28g

Spicy Buffalo Wings

Chicken wings served this way are called 'buffalo' wings, as the original recipe using Frank's original hot sauce was created in Buffalo, New York. Although I have a general mistrust of things that come in jars, I do love the smoky heat of chipotle and harissa pastes as well as Frank's hot sauce, which is spicy and sugar-free. They all add flavour and heat to chicken and all three are readily available in supermarkets. I love these with the Sweetheart Cabbage and Carrot Slaw on page 201 or the Avocado Cream on page 78. This makes a substantial meal, so perhaps enjoy this on a day when you are having other light meals.

1. You may need to cook the wings in batches. Spread the frozen chicken wings over a crisper in the drawer, then air fry at 200°C (400°F) for 10 minutes. Turn them over with tongs and cook them for a further 10 minutes, or until the internal temperature measures 75°C (167°F). Check the chicken is done by cutting the thickest piece in half and making sure there are no pink juices running from it.

2. Meanwhile, put the hot sauce in a large mixing bowl.

3. Once the chicken is cooked, tip the wings into the bowl and thoroughly coat the wings in the sauce using 2 large spoons. Spread the wings back over the crisper and return it to the air fryer for another 5 minutes.

4. Remove the wings from the air fryer and serve straight away with a side of your choice.

475g (1lb 1oz) frozen chicken wings
2 tablespoons Frank's RedHot Original sauce, or chipotle or harissa paste

Tips and tricks
Use fresh chicken wings:
Air fry at 200°C (400°F) for 15 minutes, turning halfway, or until cooked through. Coat the wings with the sauce, then cook for a further 5 minutes.

Per serving: 603kcal			
NET CARBS	FIBRE	PROTEIN	FAT
0g	0g	56g	40g

Giorgio's Fried Chicken

Our son Giorgio was determined to make a crispy, fried chicken that was good for us and easy to make, instead of ordering a bucket of it loaded with a carb-heavy coating and fried in poor-quality oil.

1. Mix the chicken in a bowl with the buttermilk. Cover and leave in the refrigerator for a minimum of 30 minutes, or up to overnight.

2. In the meantime, or when you are ready to cook, prepare the coating by mixing all the dry ingredients together in a bowl.

3. To coat the chicken, dip it into the coating mixture piece by piece. Place the chicken, spaced apart, on an oiled crisper in the drawer and spray with oil. Bake at 160°C (325°F) for 10 minutes, or until the internal temperature measures 75°C (167°F). If you don't have a temperature probe, check it is done by piercing the thickest part with a skewer and making sure there are no pink juices running from it.

4. Serve hot.

Tips and tricks
Use boneless, skinless chicken thighs instead of breasts: prepare them in the same way but allow a few minutes more to cook them all the way through.

An alternative spice mixture to the coating above: use 1 teaspoon of Cajun or Creole spice mix instead of the oregano, ginger and mustard powder. Always taste the dry mix as you add the spices, as they can be salty.

300g (10½oz) boneless, skinless chicken breasts, cut into 3cm-(1¼ inch)-wide strips
2 tablespoons buttermilk or Greek yogurt
1 teaspoon dried oregano
2 teaspoons ground ginger
1 teaspoon mustard powder
30g (1oz) ground almonds or 3 tablespoons wheat bran
15g (½oz) finely grated Parmesan, Grana Padano or Italian-style hard cheese
2 teaspoons extra-virgin olive oil

Per serving with almonds: 451kcal			
NET CARBS	FIBRE	PROTEIN	FAT
2g	2g	41g	19g
Per serving with wheat bran: 281kcal			
NET CARBS	FIBRE	PROTEIN	FAT
2g	2g	38g	12g

Korean-style Chicken Wings

Our son Giorgio was determined to make low-carb, air-fried chicken, and after much trial and tribulation he succeeded! Gochujang paste is available in supermarkets. Pick the best stock cube you can find, preferably with no MSG or other additives. It best to cook this on the bottom of the drawer with nonstick baking paper, or a silicone liner if you prefer, as the chicken tends to stick to the crisper.

1. For the brine, put the salt and vinegar in a large bowl with 100ml (3½fl oz) cold water and mix until dissolved. Add the chicken wings, then cover with more cold water and mix once more. Leave in the refrigerator for at least 30 minutes and up to 1 hour while you prepare the batter.

2. Spray or brush oil over the base of the air fryer drawer or line it with a silicone liner.

3. Put 75g (2½oz) of the flour into a bowl with 75ml (2½fl oz) cold water. Crumble the stock cube into it and whisk until smooth. Put the rest of the flour into another bowl.

4. After the chicken has brined, drain it and pat dry with kitchen paper. Dust the wings in the dry flour before coating them thinly with the batter. Dust the chicken wings once more with the dry flour, and then place them carefully on the bottom of the air fryer drawer. Generously spray the chicken with oil.

5. Cook the wings at 160°C (325°F) for 8 minutes. Turn them gently with tongs and cook them at 220°C (425°F) for a further 5 minutes. Check the chicken is done by cutting the thickest piece in half and making sure there are no pink juices running from it. Or use a temperature probe to ensure the internal temperature of the thickest part of the chicken measures at least 75°C (167°F).

6. Meanwhile, put the garlic for the sauce in a frying pan with the butter over a medium-high heat and cook for a couple of minutes without burning it, then add the rest of the sauce ingredients along with 150ml (5fl oz) water. Bring to the boil for roughly 30 seconds, then switch off the heat. The sauce is ready.

7. Once the chicken wings are done, carefully place them in a dish and pour the sauce over them. Garnish with the spring onion and sesame seeds or coriander leaves, if using – the choice is yours.

For the brine
2 tablespoons salt
2 tablespoons any vinegar

For the battered chicken
780g (1lb 12oz) chicken wings
extra-virgin olive oil
150g (5½oz) chickpea flour
1 organic chicken stock cube

For the sauce
2 garlic cloves, grated
50g (1¾oz) butter
1 tablespoon gochujang paste
½ teaspoon cayenne pepper
1 tablespoon tomato purée
1 tablespoon erythritol or
   2 teaspoons honey
½ teaspoon any vinegar

To serve
1 spring onion, finely chopped
1 teaspoon sesame seeds (optional)
a few fresh coriander leaves (optional)

Per serving of wings: 523kcal			
NET CARBS	**FIBRE**	**PROTEIN**	**FAT**
19g	4g	43g	28g
Per serving of sauce with erythritol: 99kcal			
NET CARBS	**FIBRE**	**PROTEIN**	**FAT**
2g	0g	0g	10g
Per serving of sauce with honey: 106kcal			
NET CARBS	**FIBRE**	**PROTEIN**	**FAT**
4g	0g	0g	10g

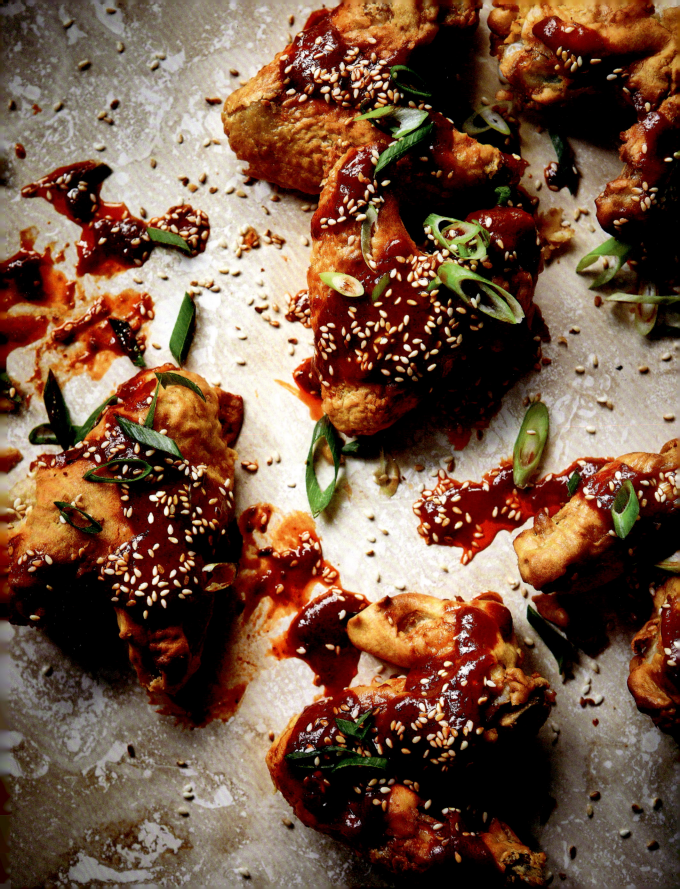

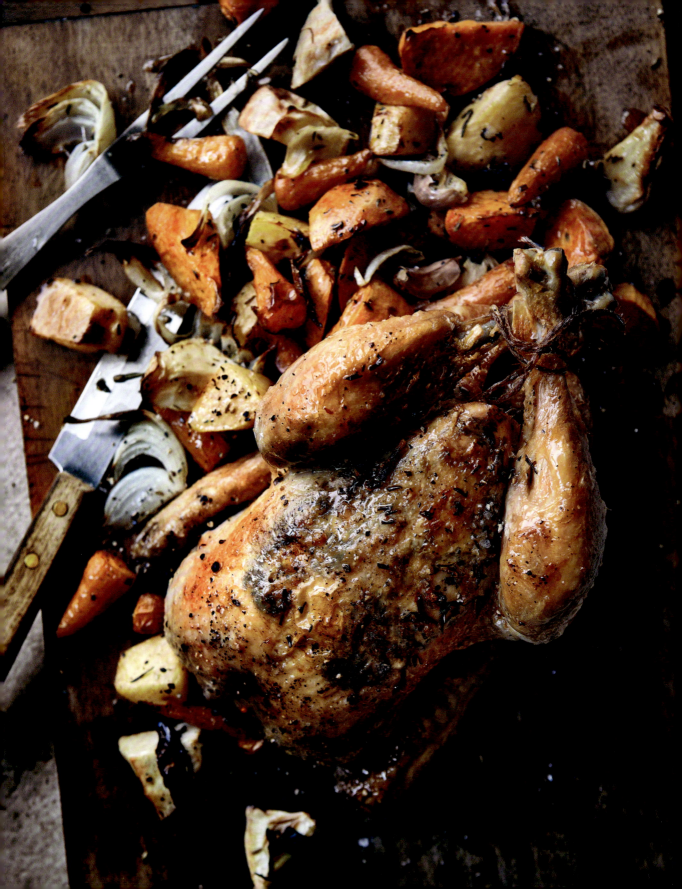

Giancarlo's Tuscan Roast Chicken

My husband, Giancarlo, loves this chicken; he cooks it how his mother made it every week in Tuscany. The chicken was flavoured with herbs that she grew in her garden and that we now have growing in ours. The incredible flavour is made by stuffing a herb paste into cuts in the flesh. We love this with a salad, but it is also good with Roasties (see page 140) or any green vegetable sides.

1. Pile the rosemary, garlic, sage, salt and plenty of pepper on a chopping board and using a cook's knife, chop them together to make a rough paste. Make 4 small cuts about 4cm (1½ inches) deep into the underneath and breasts of the chicken and force the herb paste into them.

2. Lightly season the chicken all over and then lay it, crown-side down, on a crisper in the drawer. Drizzle over the oil and air fry at 190°C (375°F) for 20 minutes. Use tongs to turn the bird over and cook again for 20 minutes, or until browned and crisp on top and cooked through. Check the chicken is done by cutting the thickest piece in half and making sure there are no pink juices running from it. Alternatively, use a temperature probe to ensure the temperature of the chicken is at least 75°C (167°F) inside the thickest part.

3. Remove the chicken from the drawer using tongs and place on a carving board. Cover loosely with tin foil and leave to rest for 15 minutes or so before serving with the juices from the drawer in a jug on the side.

3g (⅛oz) rosemary leaves
1 fat garlic clove
3g (⅛oz) sage leaves
good pinch of salt, plus extra
    for seasoning
1.2kg (2lb 10oz) whole trimmed
    chicken
2 tablespoons extra-virgin olive oil
freshly ground black pepper

Per serving: 394kcal			
NET CARBS	FIBRE	PROTEIN	FAT
0g	0g	36g	27g

Chicken Tagliata

Tagliata means 'cut' in Italian and it refers to the fact that the chicken is cut into strips while hot to allow the unctuous spicy dressing to soak in. This recipe comes from Gino Borella who was Head Chef of San Lorenzo in Knightsbridge for 30 years. Over these years, he cooked thousands of chicken breasts for so many famous people, including Princess Diana, and this was one of her favourite dishes. We love it too. It is easy, quick and so moreish. The dressing will keep for up to a week in the refrigerator.

1. Spray or brush a rack or crisper in the drawer with oil.

2. Prepare the dressing by finely chopping the rosemary leaves, chilli and garlic together on a chopping board in a pile with some salt and pepper. Mix with the olive oil and balsamic vinegar in a small bowl. Set aside.

3. Butterfly the chicken breast by cutting it three-quarters of the way through with a sharp knife along one long side, then opening it out like wings and flattening it under a piece of cellophane or strong nonstick baking paper with a meat tenderizer or the base of a small saucepan. It should be around 1cm (½ inch) thick all over to ensure it evenly cooks.

4. Season the breast with a little salt and pepper, then spray or brush with olive oil on both sides.

5. Place the breast on the rack or crisper and air fry at 200°C (400°F) for 5 minutes. Use tongs to turn it over and cook for a further 5 minutes, or until cooked through. Check the chicken is done by cutting the thickest part in half and making sure there are no pink juices running from it. Alternatively, use a temperature probe to ensure the temperature of the chicken is at least 75°C (167°F) inside the thickest part.

6. Arrange the rocket leaves and Parmesan shavings on a plate or large wooden chopping board. When the chicken is cooked, slice it into strips and transfer to the serving dish. Drizzle the dressing over and serve straight away.

extra-virgin olive oil
1 large or 2 small boneless, skinless chicken breasts (approx. 300g/10½oz total weight)
75g (2½oz) rocket leaves or watercress
10g (¼oz) Parmesan, Grana Padano or Italian-style hard cheese, shaved
salt and pepper

For the dressing
leaves from 1 rosemary sprig
½ red chilli, or to taste
1 small garlic clove
1 tablespoon extra-virgin olive oil
1 teaspoon balsamic vinegar
salt and pepper

Per serving: 293kcal			
NET CARBS	FIBRE	PROTEIN	FAT
2g	1g	37g	14g

Narinder's Chicken Tikka

Serves 6

Our friend Bob's grandmother, on a visit from India, built her own tandoor out of clay soil in the garden of Bob's suburban London family home. Her daughter Narinder, Bob's mother, grew vegetables, kept her own chickens and made this dish in the tandoor. You will be astounded by how such an authentic-seeming flavour and texture can be created in an air fryer – which like a tandoor uses dry heat and air circulation. Serve with Cauliflower Rice, Chilli Chickpeas, Garlic Naan, salad and Cucumber Raita (see pages 199, 136, 159 and 195) for a homemade Indian banquet.

1. Using either 2 drawers or a large air fryer, spray or brush a crisper with oil.

2. To make the paste, mix all the ingredients together in a large mixing bowl with plenty of pepper. Taste the paste and add more salt or spice to your liking. Add the chicken and thoroughly mix until the cubes are coated on all sides.

3. To cook the onions and chicken, you may need to work in 2 batches. Spread the onions over the prepared crisper, scatter them with seasoning and spray with oil. Cook at 200°C (400°F) for 10 minutes, shaking the drawer halfway through.

4. Tip the chicken pieces on top and spread out so they are just separated to allow them to cook and crisp on all sides. Air fry at 200°C (400°F) for 12–15 minutes, or until browned and cooked through, turning them with tongs halfway through. Check the chicken is done by cutting the thickest piece in half and making sure there are no pink juices running from it. Alternatively, use a temperature probe to ensure the temperature of the chicken is at least 75°C (167°F) inside the thickest part.

5. Serve the chicken hot with the onions and lemon wedges.

For the paste
1 fat garlic clove, finely grated, or 1 teaspoon garlic granules
25g (1oz) fresh root ginger, peeled and finely grated
1 teaspoon garam masala
1 teaspoon ground coriander
2 tablespoons tandoori spice mix, or more to taste
1 teaspoon ground turmeric
½–1 teaspoon chilli powder or chilli flakes, to taste
1 teaspoon salt
1 tablespoon extra-virgin olive oil
2 tablespoons tomato purée
100g (3½oz) Greek yogurt
freshly ground black pepper

For the chicken
1 teaspoon extra-virgin olive oil
800g (1lb 12oz) boneless, skinless chicken breasts or thighs, cut into 3cm (1¼ inch) cubes
2 onions, thinly sliced
salt and pepper
lemon wedges, to serve

Per serving: 286kcal			
NET CARBS	FIBRE	PROTEIN	FAT
5g	1g	42g	9g

Greek-inspired Chicken Salad with Halloumi Croutons

During a few trips to Thessaloniki in Northern Greece, I was inspired to serve huge salads on wooden boards for sharing. I love the Greek abundant use of vegetables and herbs. This dish is great for using up cooked chicken; or you could air fry a breast using the method in the Chicken Tagliata recipe on page 102. Add whatever vegetables you have in the refrigerator or make the Roasted Mediterranean Vegetables on page 138. I sometimes add Toasted Pumpkin Seeds (see page 137) to this, too, as they take only a few minutes in the air fryer.

1. Spray or brush a crisper in the drawer with oil.

2. Soak the spring onions in a bowl of cold water to take the strong, raw flavour away.

3. Lay all the vegetables and the chicken together or separately on your biggest wooden chopping board or in a large bowl.

4. Mix up the dressing ingredients in a small bowl and season to taste. Set aside.

5. Drain the spring onions and add these to the board with the olives.

6. Put the halloumi into a bowl, toss with the herbs and then spray with oil all over to coat. Put the cheese on the crisper and air fry at 240°C (475°F) for 3 minutes or at 200°C (400°F) for 5 minutes, or until golden brown and starting to soften, tossing the cubes in the drawer halfway through.

7. Tip the hot halloumi croutons over the salad and pour over the dressing. Scatter over the mint, if liked, and serve straight away.

extra-virgin olive oil
4 spring onions, chopped
1 red Romano or bell pepper, cored, deseeded and cut into finger-width strips
2 celery sticks, roughly chopped
½ cucumber, peeled and chopped
1 romaine heart or little gem lettuce (approx. 200g/7oz), roughly torn
300g (10½oz) cooked chicken, chopped
75g (2½oz) Kalamata olives, pitted
large handful of mint leaves, to serve (optional)

For the dressing
finely grated zest and juice of ½ lemon, plus extra zest to garnish
3 tablespoons extra-virgin olive oil
salt and pepper

For the halloumi croutons
220g (8oz) halloumi cheese, cut into 2cm (¾ inch) cubes
1 teaspoon dried oregano or thyme
1 tablespoon extra-virgin olive oil

Per serving of halloumi croutons: 181kcal			
NET CARBS	FIBRE	PROTEIN	FAT
1g	0g	13g	14g

Per serving of the whole salad: 525kcal			
NET CARBS	FIBRE	PROTEIN	FAT
9g	5g	39g	36g

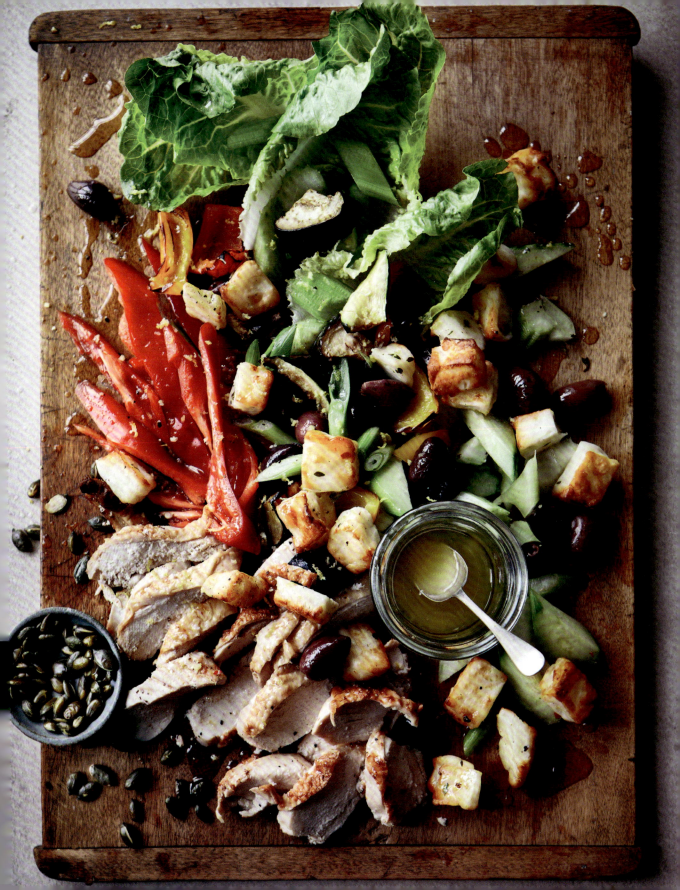

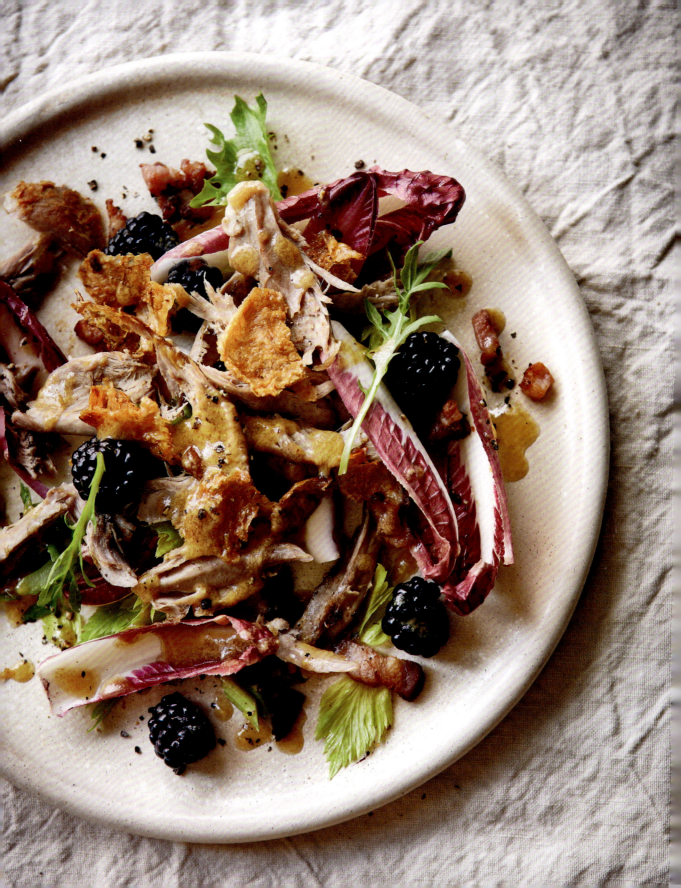

Crispy Duck, Pancetta and Blackberry Salad

This uses an old way to make a dressing from before bottles of olive oil were easily available. Hot, delicious duck and pancetta fat is used instead. This is an easy salad that can be prepared in advance, with the dressing warmed at the last minute, which is ideal if you want it as a starter for four.

1. Season the duck legs all over with salt and pepper and place on a crisper in the drawer, then air fry at 190°C (375°F) for 1 hour, or until the skin is crisp and the duck is cooked through. You will know when it is done if the meat is easy to pull away from the bone. Remove the duck legs and place on a plate, then set aside.

2. Tip the pancetta into the drawer and air fry at 200°C (400°F) for 4–5 minutes until crispy. Use tongs to remove the pancetta and set aside with the duck. Remove the crisper and taste the juices in the drawer. If they are very salty, don't use them and instead add the tablespoon of extra-virgin olive oil to the drawer. If they taste delicious (and they usually do) and if there is around a tablespoon of fat, don't add any further oil.

3. Pour the fat into a small bowl and add the mustard, vinegar, some pepper and the honey, if using. Whisk the dressing and taste, adjusting the seasoning with salt and pepper as necessary.

4. Pull the skin off the duck legs and reserve. Arrange the salad leaves and blackberries on 2 plates. Tear the duck meat from the bones and add to the salad, along with the pancetta. Divide the dressing between the plates and crumble or snip the duck skin on top. Add a twist of pepper and serve straight away.

2 duck legs
50g (1¾oz) smoked pancetta lardons or chopped smoked streaky bacon
1 tablespoon extra-virgin olive oil (optional, if needed)
1 teaspoon wholegrain or Dijon mustard
1 tablespoon red wine vinegar
1 teaspoon honey (optional)
75g (2½oz) salad leaves
50g (1¾oz) blackberries, halved if huge
salt and pepper

Per serving for 2: 334kcal			
NET CARBS	FIBRE	PROTEIN	FAT
6g	3g	32g	19g
Per serving for 4: 334kcal			
NET CARBS	FIBRE	PROTEIN	FAT
3g	1g	16g	10g

Simple Steak

It is always a good idea to warm steak up to room temperature for 30 minutes before you start to cook. This ensures a warm centre, even if you like it rare. I like this with watercress and Fries (see page 141), but any green vegetable would be ideal.

Most chefs use their fingers to tell when a steak is done by pressing the top of it while it is still in the pan. You can compare the feeling to various parts of your hand, using this guide:

Press the thumb and index finger of one hand together and, with the index finger of the other hand, prod the soft fleshy area between the base of your thumb and the base of your hand. Rare steak will be soft to the touch like this. Now press your middle finger and thumb together and feel the same point at the base of your thumb. Medium-rare will feel like this. Doing the same with the third finger will feel like medium, and with the little finger, well done.

Here is my guide to cooking times, but this is not set in stone since air fryers differ:

3–4 minutes for rare, internal temperature 45°C (113°F)
6 minutes for medium-rare, internal temperature 55°C (131°F)
7 minutes for medium, internal temperature 60°C (140°F)
9 minutes for well done, internal temperature 65°C (149°F)

1. Preheat the air fryer to 200°C (400°F).

2. Pat the steak dry with kitchen paper. Season the steak generously with salt and pepper and spray both sides with olive oil. Lay the steak down on the rack or crisper in the drawer and air fry according to the timings above.

3. Remove the steak from the air fryer and set aside in a warm place to rest for around 10 minutes before serving.

1 sirloin or rib-eye steak, measuring 2cm (¾ inch) thick (approx. 220g/8oz)
1 teaspoon olive oil
salt and pepper

Tips and tricks

Garlic and rosemary butter: This is gorgeous over steak or chicken breast. Basil or thyme is great if you don't have rosemary.

Using a fork, in a small bowl mash together 1 teaspoon finely chopped rosemary leaves, 1 teaspoon finely chopped garlic (fresh or frozen), 2 teaspoons softened butter and a pinch of salt and freshly ground black pepper. As soon as the steak is done, spoon the butter on top to melt as the steak rests.

Per serving of steak: 390kcal			
NET CARBS	FIBRE	PROTEIN	FAT
0g	0g	66g	14g

Per serving of butter: 72kcal			
NET CARBS	FIBRE	PROTEIN	FAT
1g	0g	0g	8g

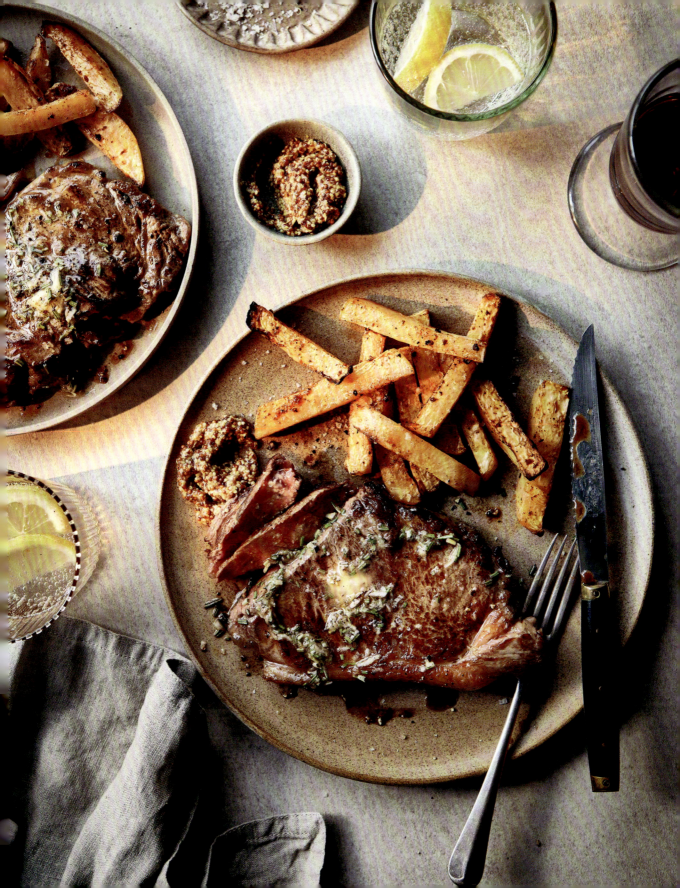

Ragú Recipes (pictured overleaf)

Quick Cheesy Mince

Serves 2

This is a delicious way to eat ragù. Simply add the cheesy topping to the mince and you have a quick and filling supper in minutes.

1. Warm the ragù in a saucepan over a medium-high heat until bubbling hot. Spoon the ragù into 1 or 2 deep ovenproof dishes to fit your air fryer. You will need at least 3cm (1¼ inches) of space above the ragù for the cheese topping to rise.

2. Beat the eggs with the cheese in a bowl and pour this over the ragù. Air fry at 180°C (350°F) for 12–15 minutes, or until the egg mixture is set and cooked.

3. Serve straight away with Mediterranean veg, any green vegetables or salad.

300g (10½oz) Tuscan Ragù (see page 203)
2 eggs
35g (1¼oz) Cheddar, smoked Cheddar or feta cheese, coarsely grated

Per serving: 414kcal			
NET CARBS	FIBRE	PROTEIN	FAT
4g	1g	29g	30g

Moussaka

Serves 2

My cheat's version of this wonderful Greek dish. I've omitted potatoes, which are often used, and made a simple, flour-free sauce.

1. Spray or brush a crisper in the drawer generously with oil.

2. Lay the aubergine slices on the oiled crisper and spray with oil. Season lightly with salt and pepper. Roast at 200°C (400°F) for 10 minutes, or until lightly browned and soft. If you have a rack, you can use this to cook a second layer at the same time, bearing in mind the ones on the rack will cook more quickly. Otherwise, roast the aubergine slices in batches. Remove from the air fryer and allow to cool briefly.

3. Meanwhile, mix together all the ingredients for the topping in a bowl so that they are well blended. Season with pepper only as the cheese is salty enough, then set aside.

4. Heat the ragù in a saucepan until it is bubbling hot, adding enough water to make it into a pourable sauce. Add the cinnamon and oregano. Spoon one-third of the ragù into a deep ovenproof dish. Don't worry if it doesn't completely cover it. Lay over one-third of the aubergine slices followed by another one-third of ragù and so on until the ragù and aubergines slices are used up.

5. Pour the topping sauce over the aubergine slices and air fry at 200°C (400°F) for 10–15 minutes, or until the cheese topping has risen and browned. Serve hot.

For the moussaka filling
extra-virgin olive oil
1 aubergine, sliced into 12 circles, approx. 1cm (½ inch) thick
300g (10½oz) Tuscan Ragù (see page 203)
½ teaspoon ground cinnamon
½ teaspoon dried oregano
salt and pepper

For the topping
15g (½oz) mature Cheddar, Parmesan, Grana Padano or Italian-style hard cheese, grated
1 egg
60g (2¼oz) full-fat Greek yogurt
½ teaspoon ground nutmeg
salt and pepper

Per serving: 424kcal			
NET CARBS	FIBRE	PROTEIN	FAT
13g	5g	27g	26g

The Diabetes Air Fryer Cookbook

Cottage Pie

Traditionally, this is made with mashed potato, but this low-carb version uses celeriac or swede mash. Each has a wonderful, slightly spicy flavour with a fraction of the carbs. Use the Tuscan Ragù on page 203; I make it in a big batch and freeze in smaller portions.

1. Bring a saucepan of water to the boil. Put the swede and/or celeriac into the pan and boil for around 25–30 minutes until tender when pierced with a knife. Drain and put into a mixing bowl.

2. Add the butter and milk and season. Mash with a potato masher or a stick blender until smooth.

3. Meanwhile, warm the ragù in a saucepan over a medium-high heat until bubbling hot. Stir in the Worcestershire sauce.

4. Pour the ragù into 1 or 2 deep ovenproof dishes. Drop spoonfuls of the mash over the top and spread it out with the back of the spoon. Use a fork to make lines in the mash. Air fry at 180°C (350°F) for 15 minutes to brown. Serve straight away with greens.

300g (10½oz) Tuscan Ragù (see page 203)
1 tablespoon Worcestershire sauce

For the mash
300g (10½oz) swede or celeriac or a mix, peeled and cut into 2cm (¾ inch) cubes
15g (½oz) butter
30ml (1fl oz) full-fat milk or double cream
salt and pepper

Per serving: 407kcal			
NET CARBS	FIBRE	PROTEIN	FAT
17g	5g	22g	26g

Lasagne with Ragù and Courgette Layers

After years of making traditional Italian lasagne from fresh pasta sheets, I love the speed of using layers of courgette ribbons instead.

1. Put the courgette in a bowl and spray with oil. Season with salt and pepper and toss through. Put the courgette into the drawer and air fry at 200°C (400°F) for 6–7 minutes, or until lightly browned in places and just softened. Tip out on to a plate lined with kitchen paper to cool and drain.

2. Meanwhile, mix together all the ingredients for the quick creamy sauce in a bowl so that they are well blended. Season with pepper only as the cheese is salty enough, then set aside.

3. Pour one-third of the ragù into a deep ovenproof dish, then lay over one-third of the courgette slices. Top with one-third of the quick creamy sauce. Repeat twice more, finishing with a layer of sauce and the cheese.

4. Cover the lasagne loosely with tin foil, tucking it underneath the dish to prevent it flying around. Bake at 160°C (325°F) for 25 minutes, then remove the tin foil and bake at 200°C (400°F) for a further 5 minutes, or until bubbling and browned. Serve hot.

1 courgette, sliced into ribbons using a vegetable peeler
extra-virgin olive oil
300g (10½oz) Tuscan Ragù (see page 203)
10g (¼oz) Parmesan, Grana Padano or Italian-style hard cheese, grated
salt and pepper

For the quick creamy sauce
35g (1¼oz) Parmesan, Grana Padano, Italian-style hard cheese or mature Cheddar cheese, grated
25ml (1fl oz) double cream
120g (4¼oz) full-fat Greek yogurt
½ teaspoon ground nutmeg
freshly ground black pepper

Per serving: 511kcal			
NET CARBS	FIBRE	PROTEIN	FAT
11g	3g	30g	37g

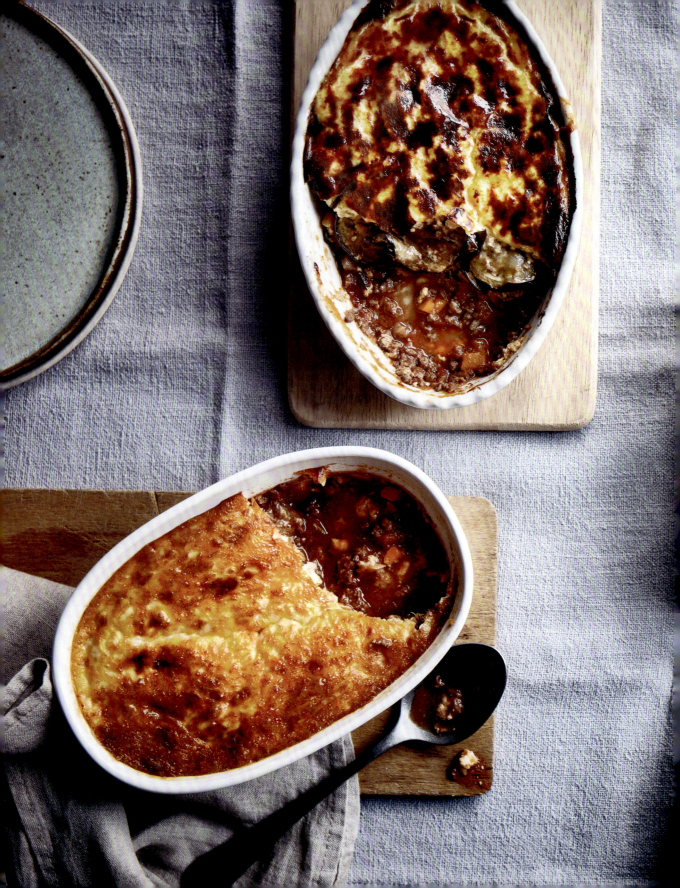

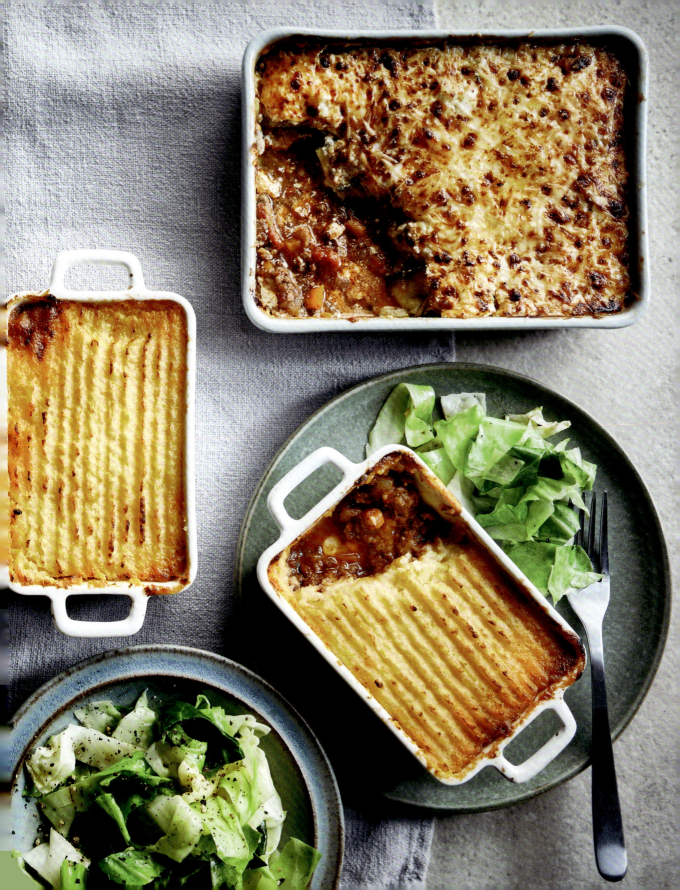

Gloria's Meatballs

Gloria is my husband's cousin from Liguria. While she was
staying with us she made this delicious meatball recipe that was a
combination of both her grandmothers' ways of making them. She
had never seen this classic dish made in an air fryer but loved the
speed and easy browning of the meatballs. In Italy, meatballs are
usually served with vegetables or greens; the idea of combining
meatballs with spaghetti is more of an American tradition.

Use defrosted frozen minced beef to keep the cost down and
swap beef for minced lamb if you prefer.

1. Bring a pan of water to the boil. Add the potato and boil for
   10–15 minutes, or until tender when pierced with a knife. Drain
   and put it into a large mixing bowl. Mash the potato and leave
   it in the bowl to cool.

2. Spray or brush a crisper in the drawer, and rack if you have one,
   with oil.

3. Add the remaining ingredients, except the tomato sauce, to the
   bowl with plenty of pepper and mix everything together with your
   hands. To check for seasoning, take a walnut-sized amount of the
   mixture, flatten the patty to 1cm (½ inch) thick and put it in the air
   fryer at 200°C (400°F) for 5 minutes, or until cooked through. Taste
   and adjust the seasoning in the mixture in the bowl with more salt
   or parsley as you like.

4. Shape the mixture into 35g (1¼oz) meatballs. Air fry them on
   the oiled crisper at 200°C (400°F) for 10 minutes, or until lightly
   browned, give them a shake to turn them halfway through cooking.
   You can use a rack above to cook more if you have one, or do them
   in batches.

5. Put the tomato sauce into a large saucepan and heat to a gentle
   bubble. Remove the meatballs from the crisper and finish cooking
   them in the tomato sauce for around 15 minutes, or until cooked
   through. Cut one open and make sure the meat is cooked and
   not pink inside. Serve with vegetable mash and sprinkled with
   extra Parmesan cheese.

150g (5½oz) potato, peeled and
   roughly chopped
extra-virgin olive oil
500g (1lb 2oz) minced beef (15% fat)
1 onion, coarsely grated
15g (½oz) parsley, or more to taste,
   finely chopped
50g (1¾oz) Parmesan, Grana Padano
   or Italian-style hard cheese, finely
   grated, plus extra to serve
1 egg
1 teaspoon salt, or more to taste
½ teaspoon dried or finely
   chopped fresh thyme
1 quantity of Classic Tomato Sauce
   (see page 196)
freshly ground black pepper

Per serving: 248kcal			
NET CARBS	FIBRE	PROTEIN	FAT
6g	1g	21g	15g

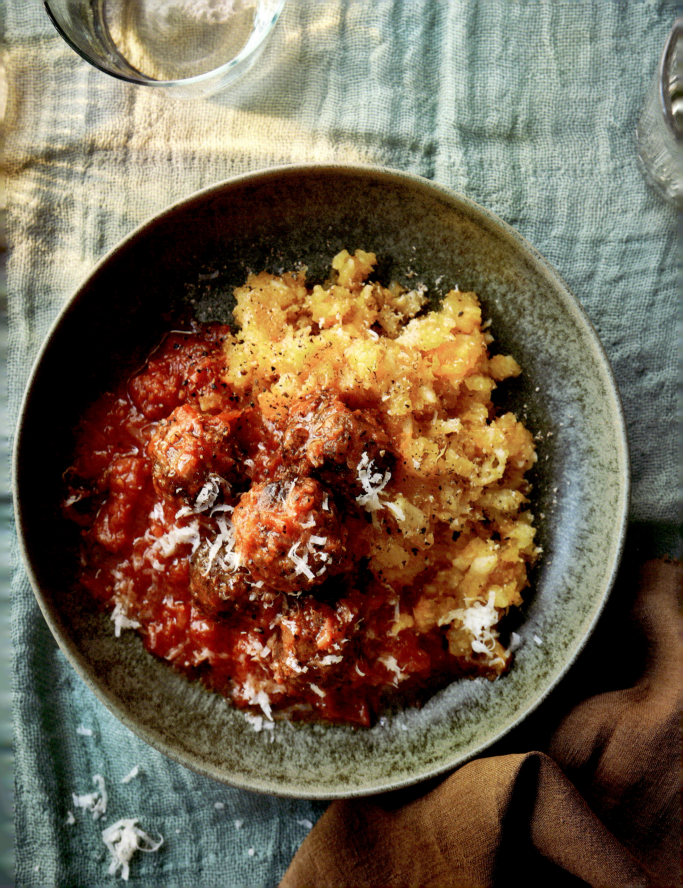

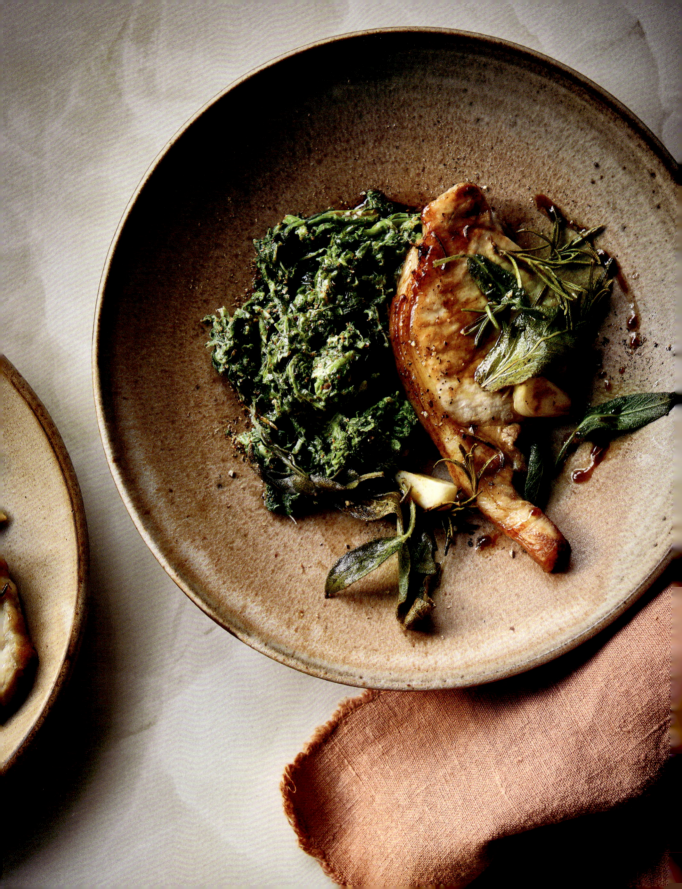

Pork Steaks with Sage and Garlic

Chops are one of my favourite inexpensive cuts of meat, but they're easy to overcook in a pan. They are great in an air fryer for quick suppers. Try this dish with Creamy Spinach with Nutmeg, Vegetable Mash or Steamed Vegetable Parcels (see pages 151, 198 and 142).

1. Spray or brush a crisper in the drawer with some of the oil. Preheat the air fryer to 200°C (400°F).

2. Dry the chops with kitchen paper and then lightly spray them with oil, then season with salt and pepper on both sides.

3. Place the herbs and garlic in 2 piles on the crisper. Lay the pork chops over the top. Air fry for 4 minutes, then turn them, leaving the herbs and garlic underneath, and cook for a further 3 minutes. Check the pork is cooked by cutting into the thickest part and making sure there are no pink juices running from it. If you have a temperature probe, check they have reached 75°C (167°F) in the middle. If it is not cooked, air fry for a few more minutes.

4. Remove from the air fryer and allow the chops to rest for 2–3 minutes on a warm plate (keep the herbs, garlic and juices in the drawer) before serving with the herbs, garlic and juices on top.

2 teaspoons extra-virgin olive oil
2 pork chops or steaks (approx. 350g/12oz total weight)
6 broad sage leaves and/or a few rosemary sprigs
2 garlic cloves, peeled and halved
salt and pepper

Per serving: 255kcal			
NET CARBS	FIBRE	PROTEIN	FAT
0g	0g	38g	10g

Sausages, Mash and Onion Gravy

This is pure comfort food and with a sweet gravy and a bowl of mashed potatoes you could soon see your glucose levels rise. Instead, make your own gravy with little to no added sweetener and choose to make one of the vegetable mashes on page 198 instead of serving it with potato mash.

1. Put the sausages in a single layer on a rack or crisper in the drawer. Air fry at 180°C (350°F) for 10–15 minutes, turning once during the cooking time, until they are cooked through. If you have a temperature probe, check they have reached 75°C (167°F) in the middle.

2. Serve with the mash and a jug of onion gravy on the side.

4 sausages
½ quantity of Vegetable Mash of your choice (see page 198), warm
⅓ quantity of Onion Gravy (see page 197), warm

Tips and tricks

Frozen sausages: If using frozen sausages, air fry them (separately or frozen together) on a rack at 180°C (350°F) for 3 minutes to defrost. Spread them out on the rack and continue to cook at 180°C (350°F) for 10–15 minutes, turning once halfway through.

Per serving of 2 sausages: 339kcal			
NET CARBS	FIBRE	PROTEIN	FAT
0g	0g	23g	28g

Lamb Chops
with Rosemary and Lemon Zest

Quickly cooking lamb steaks is wonderful for a supper in a hurry.
Serve with My Perfect Green Salad with Fresh Herbs and Vinaigrette
(see page 200) or any of the green vegetable sides in the book.

1. Preheat the air fryer to 200°C (400°F).

2. To cook the lamb, put the steaks into a bowl and spray or drizzle
   with the oil. Season on both sides and scatter over the rosemary
   and lemon zest.

3. Place the lamb on a crisper in the drawer and air fry until done
   to your liking, turning the chops halfway through. For rare allow
   4–6 minutes, for medium-rare allow 7–8 minutes and for well-
   done allow 10 minutes.

4. When the lamb is cooked to your liking, remove it from the drawer
   and let it rest in a warm place for 5–10 minutes. Serve.

500g (1lb 2oz) lamb (leg) steaks
    or 1 rack of lamb separated into
    8 cutlets
2 teaspoons extra-virgin olive oil
1 teaspoon finely chopped rosemary
finely grated zest of ½ lemon
salt and pepper

Tips and tricks
Frozen steaks/cutlets: To
cook frozen lamb steaks/cutlets,
air fry on an oiled crisper at
190°C (375°F) until soft to the
touch and thoroughly defrosted.
Depending on the thickness
of the lamb steaks/cutlets, this
can take anywhere between
10–20 minutes. Then cook
as above.

Per serving: 215kcal			
NET CARBS	FIBRE	PROTEIN	FAT
0g	0g	25g	13g

Tanzeela's Lamb Kebabs with Coriander Chutney

Our friend Habib was raving one day about his wife Tanzeela's kebabs and how quickly they cook in their air fryer. My ears pricked up (as I am always on the hunt for new recipes) and I asked for the recipe. With a little adjustment for low-carb cooking, here is a wonderful and easy recipe for kebabs which I like to serve with a coriander chutney. My advice would be to taste your green chillies before adding them to either dish, as they can be deceptively hot or mild. Serve this with Turkish Chopped Salad or Cauliflower Rice (see pages 201 and 199)

1. You will need 6 metal or wooden skewers to fit your air fryer. If using wooden skewers, soak them for at least 15 minutes in cold water first.

2. Spray or brush a crisper in the drawer with some of the oil.

3. Place all the ingredients, apart from the rest of the oil, along with plenty of pepper into a bowl, then mix thoroughly with your hands until the mixture is very well combined. Shape the mixture around the skewers into logs around 3cm (1¼ inches) across and 18cm (7 inches) long. Alternatively, make the kebab shapes without using the skewers.

4. Working in batches if needed, depending on the size of your air fryer, lay the kebabs on a crisper in the drawer and spray or brush them with the rest of the oil. Air fry the kebabs at 220°C (425°F) for 8 minutes, turning them after 5 minutes or whenever they look browned and are sizzling. Check the meat is cooked through by cutting into the thickest part of a kebab and making sure it isn't pink inside.

5. While the kebabs are cooking, make the chutney. Put all the ingredients for the coriander chutney, except the pepper, in a blender or food processor and whizz until blended, adding up to 100ml (3½fl oz) cold water to form a smooth, spoonable dip. Any leftovers will keep in a jar in the refrigerator for up to 3 days.

6. Finish the coriander chutney with a good grind of black pepper, then serve the kebabs hot with lemon wedges, little gem lettuce and sprinkling of dill.

Per kebab with chutney: 263kcal			
NET CARBS	FIBRE	PROTEIN	FAT
3g	1g	16g	20g

For the kebabs

500g (1lb 2oz) minced lamb or mutton (around 20% fat)
½ teaspoon salt
1 teaspoon ground coriander
1 teaspoon ground cumin
1 teaspoon chaat masala or curry powder
1 tablespoon lemon juice
1 tablespoon finely chopped hot green chilli or good pinch of chilli flakes
2 tablespoons finely chopped mint
2 heaped tablespoons finely chopped fresh coriander
5 spring onions, finely chopped
2 tablespoons chickpea flour
2 teaspoons extra-virgin olive oil
freshly ground black pepper

For the coriander chutney

15g (½oz) fresh coriander
15g (½oz) mint
2 teaspoons lemon juice
pinch of salt
½–1 green chilli, deseeded and roughly chopped, added according to strength
15g (½oz) fresh root ginger, peeled and roughly chopped
5 tablespoons Greek yogurt
1 teaspoon chaat masala or curry powder
1 teaspoon ground cumin
freshly ground black pepper

To serve

lemon wedges
little gem lettuce, separated into leaves
dill, to garnish

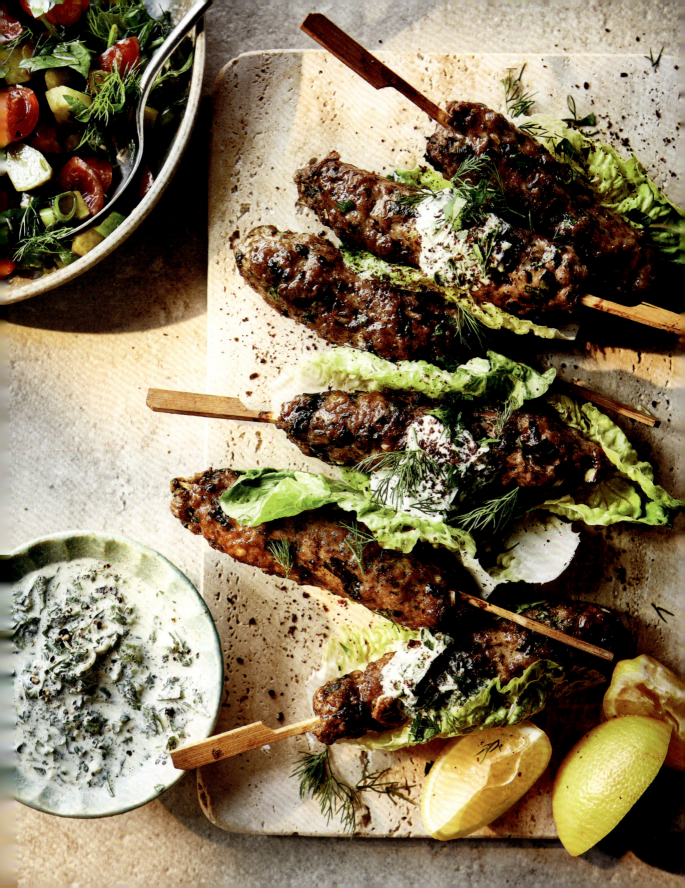

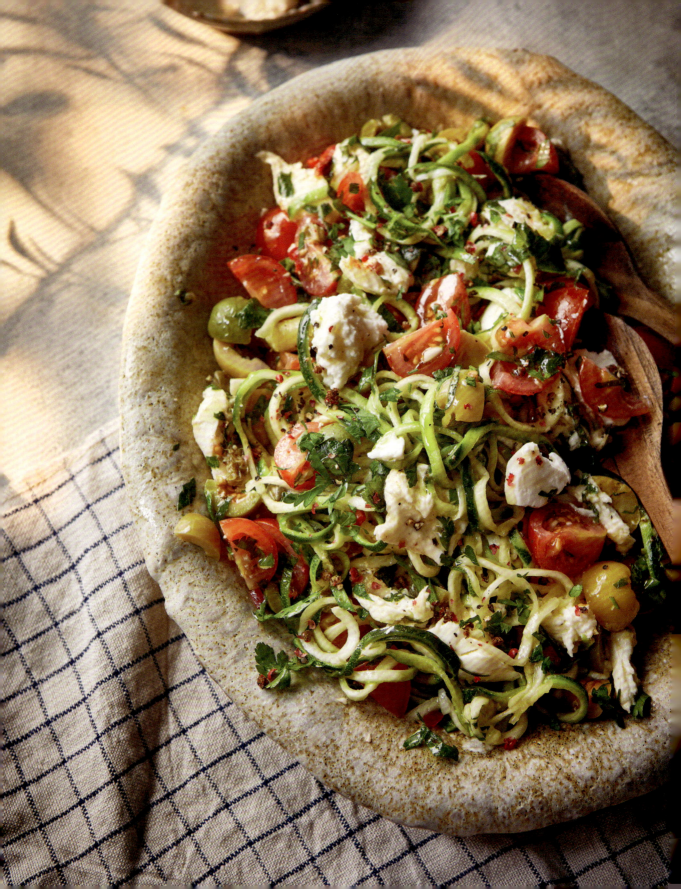

Courgetti with Roman Raw Sauce

A version of this rainbow-coloured sauce was served to us in Rome years ago and we have been making it ever since. We love the way Romans often serve cold ricotta over hot pasta or in this case hot courgetti. To bump up the protein, serve this with a low-carb bread roll (see page 156) to mop up the juices.

1. Mix all the ingredients for the sauce, except the mozzarella and ricotta, together in a large serving bowl, seasoning with salt and pepper. Set aside while you make the courgetti.

2. To make the courgetti, put the courgette(s) through a spiralizer on the finer cutter to form long strands like tagliolini. Use scissors to cut them into manageable lengths to wrap around a fork when eating. Drop them into a bowl and add the oil, garlic and some salt and pepper. Toss them through, then tip them into the drawer of the air fryer and roast at 200°C (400°F) for 4 minutes, or until they have just begun to collapse and brown.

3. Use tongs to remove them from the drawer, discarding any water left in the drawer and stir into the sauce, along with the mozzarella. Divide between 4 bowls and top with spoonfuls of ricotta. Serve straight away.

For the sauce
200g (7oz) cherry tomatoes, quartered
1 small garlic clove, finely chopped
3 tablespoons finely chopped parsley
3 tablespoons finely chopped basil
20g (¾oz) capers, rinsed well
80g (2¾oz) pitted green olives, quartered
½ hot red chilli, finely chopped, or pinch of chilli flakes
2 tablespoons extra-virgin olive oil
125g (4½oz) buffalo mozzarella cheese, roughly torn
salt and pepper
100g (3½oz) ricotta cheese, to serve

For the courgetti
1 large or 2 small courgettes
1 teaspoon extra-virgin olive oil
1 small garlic clove, roughly chopped
salt and pepper

Per serving of courgetti: 25kcal			
NET CARBS	FIBRE	PROTEIN	FAT
3g	1g	1g	1g
Per serving of sauce with ricotta: 202kcal			
NET CARBS	FIBRE	PROTEIN	FAT
5g	1g	8g	17g

Roast Tomato Sauce

When tomatoes are in season, ripe and bursting with flavour, it's worth making your own sauce in around 30 minutes in small batches in the air fryer. At other times, canned Italian plum tomatoes are ideal. This sauce can be made with large, small or cherry tomatoes or a mix of them all. Serve the sauce with the Stuffed Courgettes with Ricotta and Mint (see page 126), just like a tomato passata (sieved tomatoes), with eggs or tofu for a protein-packed meal.

1. Put the tomatoes, 2 of the basil sprigs and the onion into the air fryer drawer (with no rack) or into a silicone dish with no holes. Air fry at 170°C (340°F) for 20–25 minutes, or until the tomatoes have released their juices and softened, shaking the drawer twice during the cooking time and making sure the onion and basil are under the tomatoes, so they don't burn.

2. When the tomatoes are soft, remove the basil sprigs, then use a stick blender in the drawer, or transfer the mixture to a blender, and whizz up the tomatoes, skins and all, until you have a smooth sauce.

3. Put the olive oil and garlic cloves together in a clean drawer or silicone dish,, then air fry at 200°C (400°F) for a couple of minutes until you smell garlic. Add the tomato mixture, the remaining basil and a splash of water to dilute the sauce to a thick pouring consistency. Cook for 5 minutes until the mixture is hot.

4. Taste and season accordingly. Now it is ready to use straight away or decant into a container, then cool and store in the refrigerator for up to 5 days or freeze for up to 3 months. Defrost before use.

1kg (2lb 4oz) ripe and very red tomatoes, quartered
4 basil sprigs (10 leaves)
1 small onion, quartered and separated into petals
4 tablespoons extra-virgin olive oil
2 garlic cloves, peeled and lightly crushed using the flat of a knife
salt and pepper

Tips and tricks

Protein-packed vegan tomato sauce: Per serving, put 150g (5½oz) cooked tomato sauce and 200g (7oz) silken tofu into a blender and whizz until smooth. Heat in the microwave or a small pan until hot, then mix with hot cabbage ribbons or other low-carb veggies of your choice.

Eggs in tomato sauce: Per serving, put 150g (5½oz) cooked tomato sauce into a small frying pan over a medium heat. When the sauce is hot, crack in 2 eggs and season them. Put a lid on the pan and cook for 5–7 minutes, or until the eggs are cooked to your liking. Serve in a bowl on its own or with low-carb bread.

Per serving: 174kcal			
NET CARBS	FIBRE	PROTEIN	FAT
9g	3g	3g	14g
Per serving with tofu (not including veggies): 298kcal			
NET CARBS	FIBRE	PROTEIN	FAT
13g	4g	16g	19g
Per serving with 2 eggs: 348kcal			
NET CARBS	FIBRE	PROTEIN	FAT
10g	3g	17g	26g

Roast Cauliflower
with Tahini Mushrooms and Thyme

Tahini is an amazing match for mushrooms, adding a nutty flavour and a creamy texture. For extra protein, add the Chilli Chickpeas from page 126 or a couple of poached or fried eggs (see page 42). An air fryer is great for roasting cauliflower or broccoli florets.

1. Spray or brush a crisper in the drawer with oil.

2. Put the cauliflower into a bowl and add the oil and thyme, then season. Use your hands to toss them together to make sure the florets are coated in oil. Lay the florets on the crisper. Roast them at 180°C (350°F) for 15 minutes, shaking the drawer twice during cooking, until tender when pierced with a knife.

3. Meanwhile (if you have 2 drawers, or afterward if you don't), put the mushrooms into the drawer or a silicone liner and spray or drizzle with the oil or melted butter as you toss them around with a spatula. Add some salt, plenty of pepper, the garlic and herb sprig and toss them again. Air fry at 200°C (400°F) for 8 minutes, moving and tossing them once halfway through. They are done when they are just soft and lightly browned.

4. Stir in the tahini with a silicone spatula and return the drawer to the air fryer to keep them warm.

5. Cut away the tough large stems from the reserved cauliflower leaves, put them into a bowl with a spray of olive oil and a little pepper and salt. Rub the oil into the leaves and place them on the crisper. Cook these in the air fryer at 200°C (400°F) for 4–5 minutes until crisp.

6. When the cauliflower is done, tip it from the drawer into 2 warm serving bowls. Pour the mushrooms over the cauliflower with the roast cauliflower leaves around the edge. Add the herbs, if using, and then serve.

1 small cauliflower (approx. 400g/14oz), cut into bite-sized florets, leaves reserved
2 tablespoons extra-virgin olive oil, plus extra for greasing and the cauli leaves
2 teaspoons chopped fresh or dried thyme, rosemary or sage leaves
salt and pepper

For the mushrooms
300g (10½oz) mushrooms, trimmed and roughly sliced
1 tablespoon extra-virgin olive oil or melted butter
1 garlic clove, peeled and lightly crushed using the flat of a knife
1 rosemary or thyme sprig, plus extra finely chopped leaves to serve (optional)
3 tablespoons tahini
salt and pepper

Per serving: 395kcal			
NET CARBS	FIBRE	PROTEIN	FAT
12g	8g	12g	33g

Stuffed Courgettes with Ricotta and Mint

Serves 2

This beautiful dish is perfect for a light lunch or would serve four as a starter. To bump up the protein, serve this with low-carb bread rolls (see page 156) or finish your meal with some Greek yogurt and berries. These also make a summery and delightful meal with the Roast Tomato Sauce on page 124.

1. Use a spoon to carefully scoop out the insides of the courgettes (keep the insides for later) leaving a boat-shaped shell of just under 1cm (½ inch) thick, being careful not to make any holes. Put the courgette halves on a crisper in the drawer and air fry at 200°C (400°F) for 10 minutes.

2. Meanwhile, mix the ricotta, egg, cheese, mint and some seasoning together in a bowl. When the courgettes are just tender and starting to lightly brown, remove them from the drawer and divide the filling between them.

3. Put the crisper into the drawer and place the courgettes on top, packed together. Drop the pine nuts evenly on top. Brush with 2 teaspoons of oil. Air fry for 8–10 minutes until lightly browned, then set the stuffed courgettes aside and keep warm.

4. Finely chop the courgette insides and mix these in a bowl with the remaining teaspoon of the oil, the onion, tomatoes and some seasoning. Remove the crisper from the air fryer, then tip the mixture into the drawer, or into an ovenproof dish, and air fry at 200°C (400°F) for 10 minutes until soft. Toss twice during the cooking time.

5. Divide the chopped courgette mixture between 2 plates, or 1 large serving plate, and arrange the stuffed courgette halves on top. Garnish with mint leaves and a swirl of olive oil.

2 courgettes (approx. 400g/14oz), halved lengthways
150g (5½oz) ricotta cheese
1 egg, beaten
20g (¾oz) Cheddar or other hard cheese, finely grated
15–20 mint leaves, chopped, or 1 heaped teaspoon dried mint, plus extra chopped leaves to garnish
25g (1oz) pinenuts or other nuts, roughly chopped
1 tablespoon extra-virgin olive oil, plus extra for drizzling
1 small onion, finely chopped
10 cherry tomatoes, halved
salt and pepper

Per serving: 362kcal			
NET CARBS	FIBRE	PROTEIN	FAT
13g	4g	16g	27g

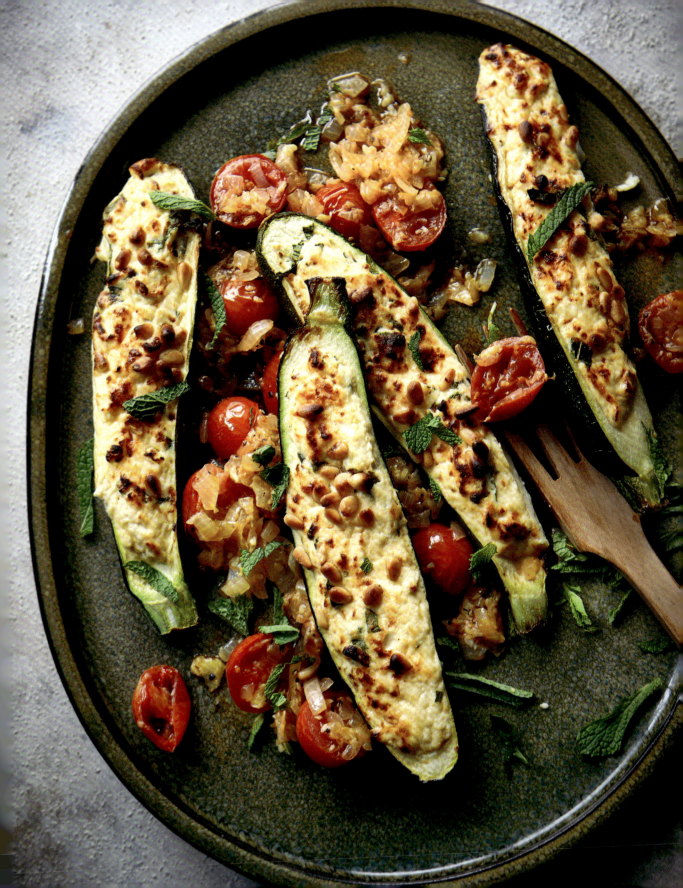

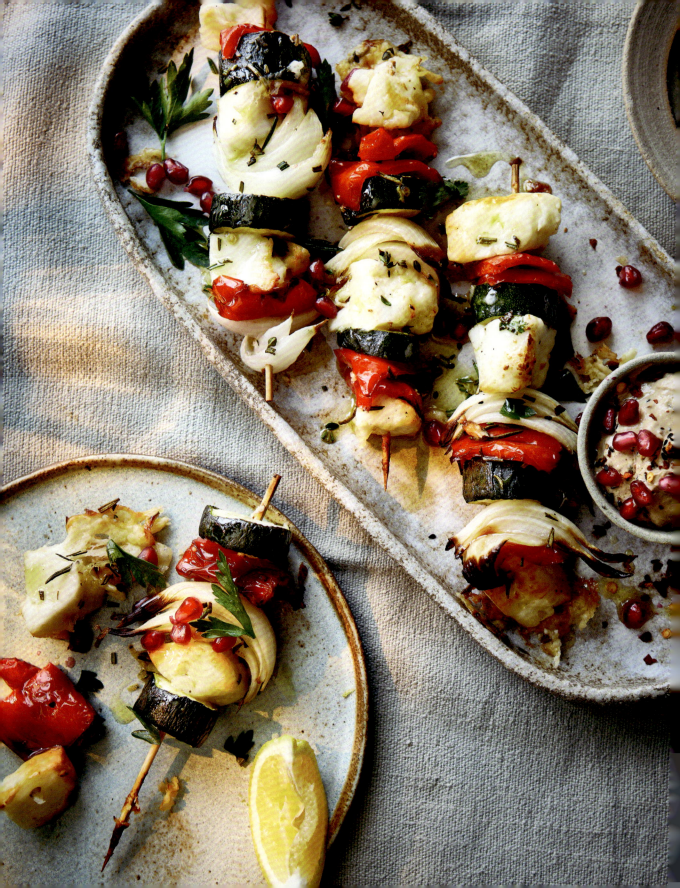

Halloumi and Vegetable Skewers with Giorgio's Chilli Sauce

Giorgio is our son and he loves spicy foods. He made up this sauce and says to 'go for it with the chilli', as the kefir cools it down. Do halve the recipe for a small portion, but we love to put the sauce into a jar; it will keep in the refrigerator for up to a week, though it always gets used up, as it goes so well with halloumi, fried chicken, veggie fries or salad. Use whatever veggies you have in the refrigerator for these skewers; small mushrooms or thin slices of aubergine work well instead of the pepper and courgette.

1. You will need 4 wooden or metal skewers. If using wooden skewers, soak them in cold water for at least 15 minutes.

2. Put 1 tablespoon of the oil, the lemon juice, the salt and plenty of pepper into a bowl and mix thoroughly.

3. Pull the onion wedges into petals and put them into the bowl with the rest of the vegetables. Add the remaining ingredients, except the rest of the oil, and gently toss through, being careful not to break up the halloumi.

4. Put a crisper into the drawer and spray or brush with the remaining oil. Preheat the air fryer to 200°C (400°F).

5. Thread the ingredients alternately on to the skewers and lay them on the oiled crisper. Cook for 3 minutes, or until the cheese is browned, then turn the skewers with tongs. Take a look at the underside; if it is equally browned, remove them from the air fryer, if not, turn them and then continue to cook for 2 minutes.

6. Serve the skewers on plates with Giorgio's chilli sauce, alongside the lemon wedges, pomegranate seeds and herbs, if using.

5 teaspoons extra-virgin olive oil
finely grated zest of ½ lemon
1 tablespoon lemon juice
pinch of salt
1 small onion, cut into 3cm (1¼ inch) wedges
1 Romano red pepper, cored, deseeded and cut into 3cm (1¼-inch) cubes
1 small courgette, cut into 1cm (½ inch) slices
approx. 225g (8oz) halloumi cheese, cut into 2–3cm (¾–1¼ inch) cubes
2 teaspoons finely chopped rosemary or thyme or dried oregano
freshly ground black pepper

To serve
Giorgio's Chilli Sauce (see page 202)
lemon wedges
small handful of fresh parsley or coriander, leaves coarsely chopped, stems finely chopped (optional)
pomegranate seeds

Per serving: 431kcal			
NET CARBS	FIBRE	PROTEIN	FAT
9g	3g	23g	33g

Aubergine Parmigiana

This classic Italian recipe is inherently low-carb; however, the aubergines are often coated in flour or breadcrumbs and then deep-fried. We were shown this lighter and simpler version with smoked cheese and roast aubergines in Amalfi and absolutely loved it!

   Smoked scamorza (an Italian cheese available from most supermarkets) melts and tastes amazing, but if you can't find it, use mozzarella instead. Share the dish for lunch or dinner with a salad or green vegetables. Alternatively, cook in two small ovenproof dishes and serve one each. The recipe freezes well, so you could cook double, wrap the extra dish(es) in tin foil and freeze for another day (for up to 3 months). Defrost in the refrigerator overnight before cooking.

1. Spray or brush a crisper in the drawer generously with oil. Working in batches, if needed, lay the slices of aubergine on it and spray with oil. Season lightly with salt and pepper. Roast the aubergine slices at 200°C (400°F) for 10 minutes, or until lightly browned and soft. If you have a rack, you can use this to cook a second layer at the same time, bearing in mind the ones on the rack will cook more quickly.

2. Remove from the air fryer and allow to cool briefly. Pour one-third of the passata into an ovenproof dish, then lay over one-third of the aubergine. Top with one-third of each cheese and one-third of the basil leaves. Repeat twice more until the ingredients are used up.

3. Cover the dish with tin foil and bake at 160°C (325°F) for 25 minutes. Remove the tin foil and bake at 200°C (400°F) for a further 5 minutes, or until bubbling and brown. Serve hot garnished with basil leaves and a good grind of pepper.

extra-virgin olive oil
1 aubergine, cut into 1cm- (½ inch)-thick circles
200g (7oz) tomato passata (sieved tomatoes) or homemade tomato sauce (see page 196 for Classic Tomato Sauce and page 124 for Roast Tomato Sauce)
130g (4½oz) smoked scamorza or mozzarella cheese, coarsely grated or cut or torn into 5mm (¼ inch) slices
15g (½oz) Parmesan, Grana Padano or vegetarian Italian-style hard cheese, finely grated
8–10 broad basil leaves, plus extra to garnish
salt and pepper

Per serving: 363kcal			
NET CARBS	FIBRE	PROTEIN	FAT
19g	7g	19g	23g

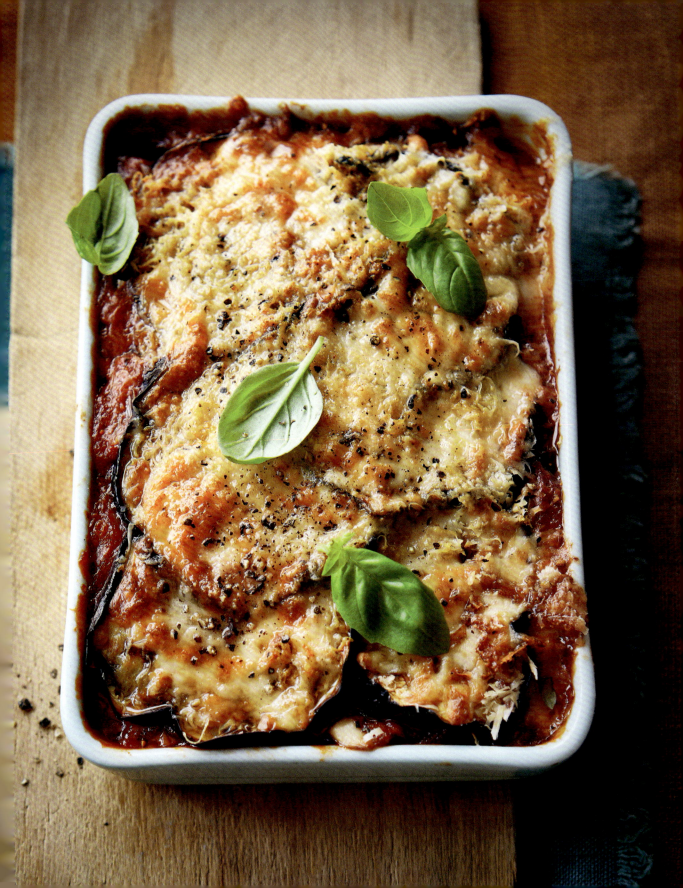

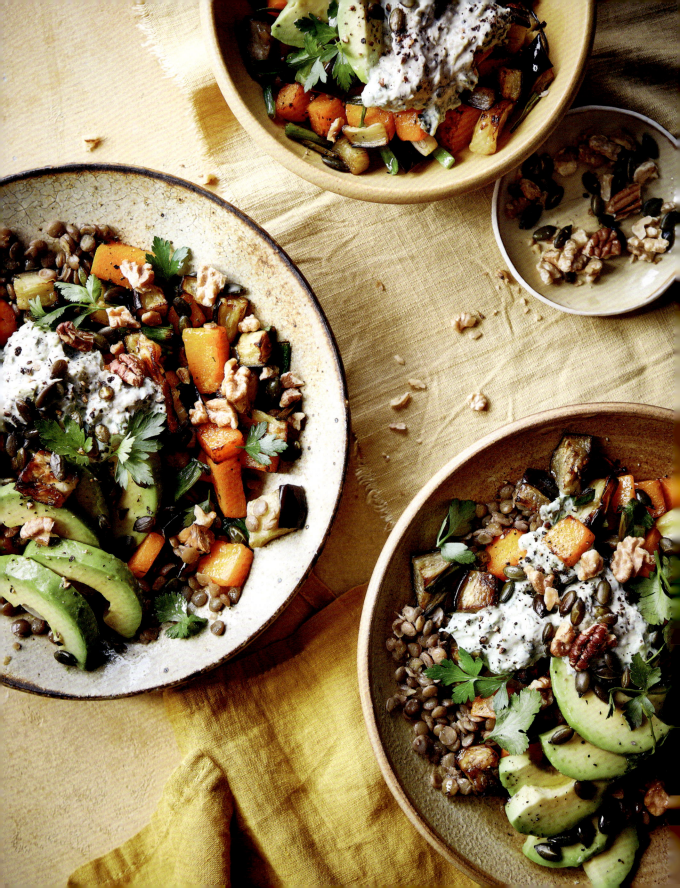

Roast Aubergine, Squash and Lentil Bowl

Serves 2

This vibrant vegan or vegetarian salad is easily made in around 30 minutes and provides enough protein while still being moderately low carb. The dressing can be made with silken tofu for vegan protein or, if you prefer, with thick Greek yogurt instead of the tofu. Adding boiled eggs gives further protein, too, if you are vegetarian. And for a bigger meal, add a handful of salad leaves.

1. Bring a pan of water to the boil. Add the lentils and boil for 25 minutes until tender, then drain.

2. Meanwhile, put the vegetables into a mixing bowl and season. Spray or drizzle with the oil and use a spoon or your hands to toss the vegetables to evenly coat.

3. Tip the vegetables on to a crisper in the drawer and spread out in a single layer. Air fry at 200°C (400°F) for 8 minutes, tossing once during cooking. Remove the spring onions, divide between 2 serving bowls and set aside.

4. Cook the remaining vegetables for a further 8 minutes until lightly browned and tender, then transfer them to the serving bowls.

5. Meanwhile, make the dressing according to the recipe below and then pour it over the salad.

6. Scatter the peanuts over the vegetables. Add the cooked lentils to the bowls, along with the avocado. Scatter with the coriander or parsley, then serve.

Coriander and Chilli Dressing

1. Make the dressing by whizzing all the ingredients together with 1 tablespoon water in a small food processor or using a stick blender in a bowl. Taste and adjust the seasoning or chilli to taste.

2. Store in the refrigerator until serving; it will keep in a sealed jar for up to 4 days.

100g (3½oz) dried green lentils, washed
1 small aubergine, cut into 3cm (1¼ inch) cubes
4 spring onions or 1 shallot, cut into 1cm (½ inch) slices or wedges
125g (4½oz) butternut squash flesh, cut into 3cm (1¼ inch) cubes
1 tablespoon extra-virgin olive oil
1 quantity of dressing (see below)
25g (1oz) roasted peanuts or other nuts, roughly chopped, and/or Toasted Pumpkin Seeds (see page 137)
flesh of 1 ripe avocado, sliced
salt and pepper
a few fresh coriander or parsley leaves, to serve

For the coriander and chilli dressing
12g (½oz) fresh coriander or a mix of mint, dill, chives, parsley or celery leaves
1 tablespoon extra-virgin olive oil
2 teaspoons lemon juice
¼–½ green or red chilli, or to taste, or pinch of chilli flakes
1 small garlic clove, peeled
100g (3½oz) silken tofu
salt and pepper

Per serving of roast aubergine, squash and lentil bowl: 427kcal			
NET CARBS	FIBRE	PROTEIN	FAT
29g	19g	14g	24g

Per serving of coriander and chilli dressing: 93kcal			
NET CARBS	FIBRE	PROTEIN	FAT
2g	0g	4g	8g

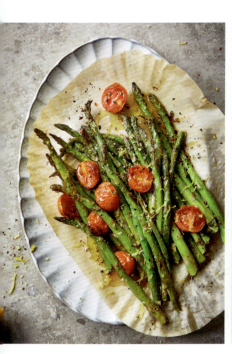
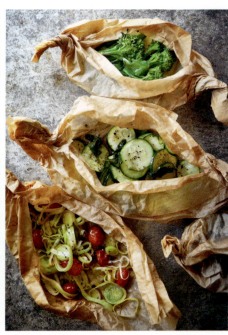
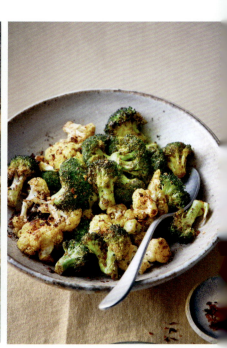

VEG SIDES

Crispy Chickpeas

Using chickpeas can be a great way to add texture and a little vegan protein to dishes; although in a 400g (14oz) can there is still only 16g protein (and the net carbs are 32g), so don't let anyone fool you into thinking they are 'loaded with protein' compared to chicken. Keep the aquafaba (the water from the can) for the Spicy Seed Crunch recipe opposite.

1. Preheat the air fryer to 200°C (400°F).

2. Drain the chickpeas well, then dry them thoroughly between 2 pieces of kitchen paper. Toss in a bowl with the olive oil, rosemary and cheese. Put them in a single layer on a crisper in the drawer and air fry for 12–15 minutes, shaking twice during cooking.

3. When the chickpeas are crispy and lightly browned, tip them on to a plate to cool. Add the salt, or to taste as necessary, and toss gently to mix. When cool, store in a jar for up to 3 days.

400g (14oz) can chickpeas
    (240g/8½oz drained weight)
1 tablespoon extra-virgin olive oil
2 tablespoons finely chopped
    rosemary leaves
3 tablespoons finely grated
    Parmesan, Grana Padano
    or vegetarian Italian-style
    hard cheese
½ teaspoon salt, or to taste

Tips and tricks
Chilli chickpeas: Follow the recipe above but instead of the rosemary and cheese, add the following spices:

½ teaspoon ground coriander
½ teaspoon ground cumin
½ teaspoon chilli powder
½ teaspoon garam masala or curry
    powder
½ teaspoon garlic granules (optional)

Per serving: 89kcal			
NET CARBS	FIBRE	PROTEIN	FAT
7g	3g	4g	4g

Spicy Seed Crunch

You can use a variety of seeds in this, but do include pumpkin and hemp, as they have the most protein. All contain healthy fats but are also high in calories, so make sure you don't mindlessly snack on them. They are intended to be a part of a meal rather than something eaten in between.

1. Line a crisper with a trimmed piece of nonstick baking paper (so that the sides don't flap around in the drawer).

2. Mix the seeds, tamari and spices in a mixing bowl.

3. In another bowl, whisk the egg white or aquafaba to stiff peaks. Gently fold it into the seeds.

4. Spread them over the lined crisper. Air fry at 200°C (400°F) for 5–7 minutes, or until completely dry and crisp, gently tossing the seeds halfway through to expose any wet areas but trying not to break up any clumps.

5. Tip out on to a plate to cool and dry. Store in a jar for up to 3 days.

150g (5½oz) mix of pumpkin, sunflower, hemp, sesame, linseed or chia seeds
2 teaspoons tamari or dark soy sauce
½ teaspoon ground ginger
½ teaspoon smoked paprika
½ teaspoon sweet paprika
½ teaspoon Aleppo chilli flakes
1 egg white or 35g (1¼oz) chickpea water (aquafaba)
¼ teaspoon hot ground spice (such as chilli powder or cayenne pepper)

Per serving: 147kcal			
NET CARBS	FIBRE	PROTEIN	FAT
2g	2g	8g	12g

Toasted Pumpkin Seeds

I love the crunch of pumpkin seeds in a salad or on top of a soup. They are a good source of protein too.

1. Put the seeds on the base of the drawer and scatter over a little salt. Roast at 200°C (400°F) for 3–5 minutes, or until they start to pop. Remove them as soon as this happens, otherwise they could hit the element above. Cool and store in a jar for up to 4 days.

50g (1¾oz) pumpkin seeds
salt

Per serving: 72kcal			
NET CARBS	FIBRE	PROTEIN	FAT
1g	1g	4g	6g

Roasted Mediterranean Vegetables

Serves 4

This is our staple recipe for roasting vegetables Italian style; we swap in what's in the refrigerator and garden. Add any vegetables likely to burn, such as broccoli, beans or cauliflower, halfway through the cooking time. This makes enough for four, which I cook even if there are only two of us, as I always like to have a bowl in the refrigerator for adding to salads, frittata, soups, etc. These are great as an accompaniment to meat, fish or eggs, or you could try them with a soft, creamy burrata or buffalo mozzarella and a scattering of basil.

Always tuck the herbs under the vegetables to give flavour and stop them burning, and space out the vegetables so that they all roast rather than steam.

1. Put the vegetables into a mixing bowl with the garlic and seasoning. Spray or drizzle with the oil and toss with your hands to coat the vegetables.

2. First put the herbs on a crisper in the drawer and then tip the vegetables and garlic on top, making sure they are in a single layer. You may have to do this in batches. Air fry at 200°C (400°F) for 10–15 minutes, tossing twice during cooking.

3. When the vegetables are lightly browned and tender, they are ready to serve.

Tips and tricks
Fry either of these (below) along with the vegetables for extra protein and flavour.

Chorizo and vegetable traybake:
Add 15g protein and 3g net carbs per serving and tons of flavour by adding 100g (3½oz) cooking chorizo sausages.

Harissa tofu cubes: Add 19g vegan protein and 3g net carbs per serving by adding harissa tofu. Coat 100g (3½oz) smoked tofu, cut into 2cm (¾ inch) cubes, with 2 teaspoons of rose harissa paste and 1 teaspoon of black onion (nigella) seeds.

1 aubergine, cut into 3cm (1¼ inch) cubes
1 red or yellow pepper, cored, deseeded and cut into 3cm (1¼ inch) cubes
1 small onion, cut into 1cm (½ inch) wedges
1 courgette, cut into 1cm (½ inch) slices
2 garlic cloves, unpeeled and lightly crushed using the flat of a knife
large pinch of salt
1 tablespoon extra-virgin olive oil
2 rosemary, thyme or sage sprigs
freshly ground black pepper

Per serving: 97kcal			
NET CARBS	**FIBRE**	**PROTEIN**	**FAT**
11g	4g	2g	4g

The Diabetes Air Fryer Cookbook

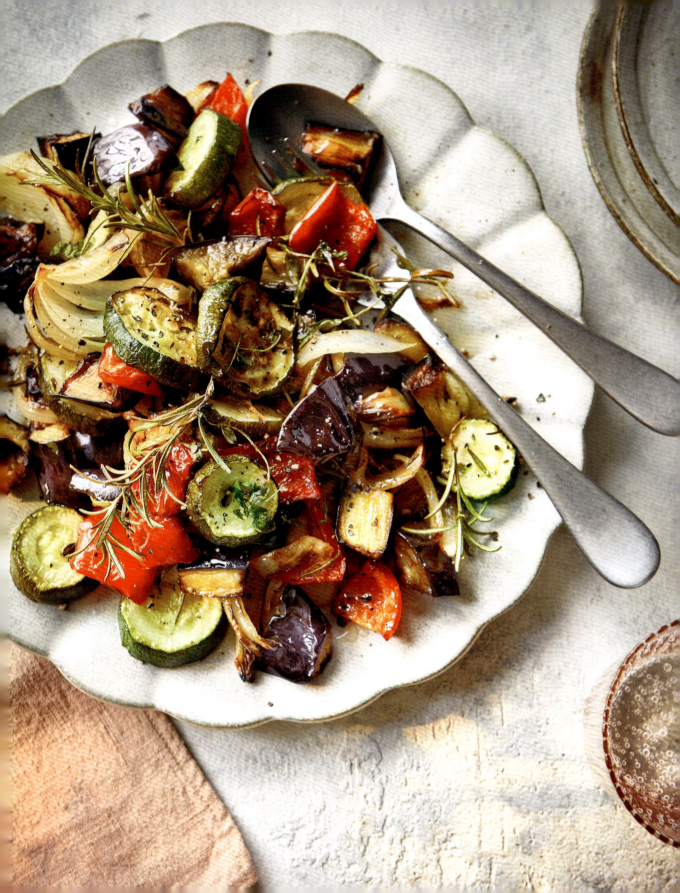

Roasties

Our family loves the flavours of these colourful roast vegetables so much that we don't miss potatoes at all! All of the peelings can be kept in the freezer and used for a homemade stock another day. The roasties are best served straight from the air fryer but can be prepared up to the point just before cooking and kept in a bowl in the refrigerator for up to a day.

1. Toss all the vegetables in a bowl with the oil, herbs, fennel seeds, garlic and some seasoning. Put them on a crisper in the drawer and roast at 190°C (375°F) for 25–30 minutes, or until just cooked through. Toss the veg mixture a couple of times during cooking to ensure even cooking. (Make sure that the herbs are tucked under the veg and that the seeds are tossed through, as light-weight foods can blow about in the air fryer.)

2. Serve straight away or keep warm, loosely covered, for up to 1 hour.

Tips and tricks
Brussels sprouts: Add a handful of halved Brussels sprouts 10 minutes into the cooking time.

500g (1lb 2oz) root vegetables such as celeriac, swede, carrots, turnips, peeled and cut into 3cm (1¼ inch) wedges or dice
1 small onion, cut into wedges
1 tablespoon extra-virgin olive oil
2 rosemary sprigs
4 large sage leaves, roughly chopped
1 teaspoon crushed fennel seeds (optional)
2 fat garlic cloves, unpeeled and crushed
salt and pepper

Per serving: 87kcal			
NET CARBS	**FIBRE**	**PROTEIN**	**FAT**
10g	4g	1g	4g

Fries

Air fryers make great fries (chips) and just because potatoes aren't on the low-carb menu, it doesn't mean you have to go without one of the world's favourite foods. Try one of the vegetables below or a mix of a few of them together for maximum flavour. Frozen sweet potatoes also work, just give them 2 more minutes to cook through. Keep the fries plain or add the spice mixture below.

1. Rinse the okra, if using, and dry with kitchen paper. However, don't mix the okra with the other vegetables, if using a mix, as they will have a separate cooking time. They will take around 10–12 minutes to cook, depending on their size.

2. If making spicy fries, mix the spices in a bowl.

3. Toss the vegetables in a bowl with the oil, some salt and the spice mixture, if using, and make sure they are evenly coated. Tip the fries on to a crisper in the drawer in a single layer. Don't overcrowd them as you need the air to circulate around them.

4. Air fry at 200°C (400°F) for around 12 minutes, tossing them halfway through by shaking the drawer or turning them with tongs. Now turn up the heat to as hot as your air fryer will go and cook for a further 3–5 minutes until golden brown and crispy. Serve straight away.

300g (10½oz) sweet potato, celeriac, carrot or swede, peeled and cut into 1cm- (½ inch)-wide fries (or bigger as you like), or okra
1 tablespoon extra-virgin olive oil
salt

For the spicy fries (optional)
1 tablespoon smoked paprika
1 teaspoon cayenne pepper
2 teaspoons garlic powder

Per serving of sweet potato fries: 115kcal			
NET CARBS	FIBRE	PROTEIN	FAT
17g	3g	2g	4g

Per serving of celeriac fries: 115kcal			
NET CARBS	FIBRE	PROTEIN	FAT
7g	3g	2g	4g

Per serving of carrot fries: 71kcal			
NET CARBS	FIBRE	PROTEIN	FAT
7g	3g	1g	4g

Per serving of swede fries: 66kcal			
NET CARBS	FIBRE	PROTEIN	FAT
6g	2g	1g	4g

Per serving of okra: 89kcal			
NET CARBS	FIBRE	PROTEIN	FAT
6g	5g	3g	4g

Steamed Vegetable Parcels

With five minutes of preparation, steamed vegetables can be transformed into a glorious array of colours, textures, flavours and excitement. In this recipe, the vegetables are cooked in paper parcels. Add herbs and spices, butter or oil, let children and fussy eaters prepare their own parcels (and name them) and generally just have fun with flavours. The juices are kept in the parcel, so go easy on the seasoning.

Here are some examples of timings and flavour suggestions. Allow a mugful of chopped vegetables and all should have salt and pepper added; enjoy these liberally as these are all low-carb veggies.

1. To make a parcel, cut a piece of nonstick baking paper around 35cm (14 inches) square.

2. Lay your chosen vegetables in the centre of the paper. Add flavours, oil or butter, and water if necessary.

3. Bring opposite corner ends of the paper up to meet each other above the food. Fold both pieces over together, with the fold around 2cm (¾ inches) wide. Fold again. Do this several times until the paper is folded around 4cm (1½ inches) above the food. Now twist each end like a sweet.

4. Place the parcels on a crisper in the drawer and air fry at 180°C (350°F) for 7–15 minutes, depending on the vegetables' density and size: more watery, soft vegetables take less time than firm carrots and the thinner you cut them the quicker they will cook. You can press the top of the parcel to feel if the veggies are tender or unwrap it and take a look. Simply re-fold the parcel and pop it back in for a couple of minutes if the vegetables are not done. Serve straight away.

Courgettes: thinly sliced, with a spray of extra-virgin olive oil and basil leaves – 7 minutes.

Leeks: thinly sliced, and whole cherry tomatoes mixed together with 10g (¼oz) butter – 8 minutes.

Savoy cabbage: shredded, with ghee, 2 tablespoons of water and pinch of cumin seeds – 8 minutes.

Cauliflower or broccoli florets: cut into bite-sized pieces, with black onion (nigella) seeds and 10g (¼oz) butter – 15 minutes.

Fennel: thinly sliced, with a few fennel seeds – 12 minutes.

Carrots and leeks: thinly sliced, with butter and chopped tarragon or parsley – 15 minutes.

Chinese cabbage: shredded, with sesame oil and sesame seeds – 5 minutes.

Sweetheart cabbage: cut into ribbons (see page 147) with 10g (¼oz) butter and 2 tablespoons of water – 12 minutes.

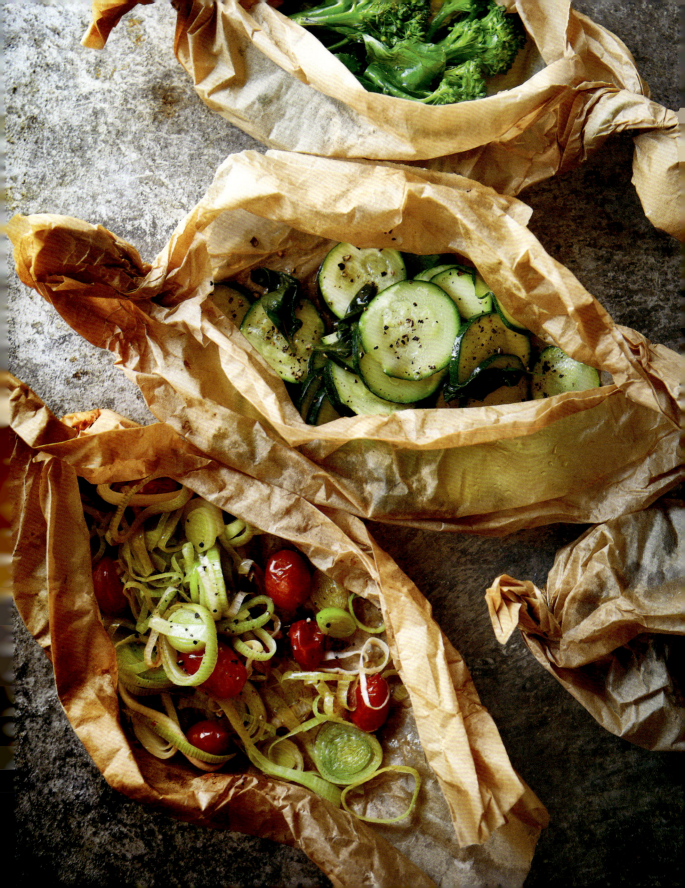

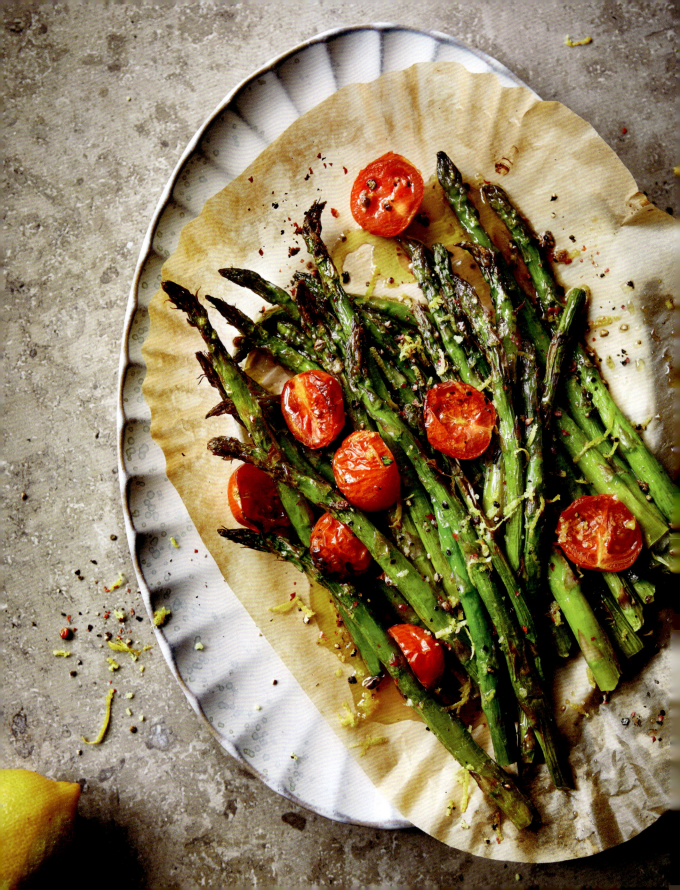

Asparagus, Tomatoes and Lemon

Asparagus is always best in season as it has more flavour if it hasn't travelled across the world to your plate. Roasting concentrates the flavour of vegetables, so the tomatoes become sweeter too. Depending on the freshness and width of your asparagus, you may need a couple of minutes less or more in the air fryer.

1. Put a baking paper liner into the drawer without a crisper.

2. Bend the asparagus spears and let them snap where the woody end meets the softer part. Discard the ends. Put the asparagus into a bowl with the cherry tomatoes, oil and seasoning. Toss together with your hands or tongs. Lay the vegetables in the liner and add the butter.

3. Air fry at 180°C (350°F) for 10–12 minutes, or until the asparagus is tender when pierced with a knife, tossing the vegetables halfway through.

4. Serve scattered with a little fresh lemon zest finely grated over the top.

240g (8½oz) asparagus
4 cherry or baby plum tomatoes, halved
2 teaspoons extra-virgin olive oil
10g (¼oz) butter
1 lemon, for zesting
salt and pepper

Per serving: 106kcal			
NET CARBS	FIBRE	PROTEIN	FAT
3g	3g	3g	9g

Smoky Roast Aubergine Moutabal

Our friend Amal Al Qahtani used to make this for our son Giorgio when she came to stay with us from Kuwait; if we weren't careful, he would eat the whole bowlful before we got a chance. At home, Amal blisters the skin of the aubergine over a flame, but we have found the air fryer works a treat, taking only 15–18 minutes to do the job.

1. Prick the aubergine all around with a sharp knife about 10 times. Put it on a crisper in the drawer and roast at 220°C (425°F) for 15–18 minutes, depending on the size, until wrinkled all over and cooked to the point where it is starting to collapse, turning it using tongs after 5 minutes.

2. Meanwhile, put the yogurt, garlic, tahini, lemon juice and seasoning into a mixing bowl and stir together.

3. Remove the aubergine from the crisper when done and set aside to cool. When cool enough to touch, cut the aubergine in half lengthways and spoon out the flesh on to a chopping board. Chop it to a pulp with a large knife and pour away any water that comes out. Put the pulp into the bowl with the remaining ingredients. Stir to combine and taste for seasoning and lemon.

4. Transfer the moutabal to a serving bowl and drizzle over the oil. Dust it with paprika or sumac and serve. The dip will keep, covered, in the refrigerator for up to a day or 2 but always garnish just before serving.

For the moutabal
1 small aubergine
1 tablespoon Greek yogurt
1 small garlic clove, grated or finely diced
2 tablespoons tahini
2 teaspoons lemon juice, or more to taste
salt and pepper

To serve
1 teaspoon extra-virgin olive oil
½ teaspoon paprika or sumac (optional)

Per serving: 117kcal			
NET CARBS	FIBRE	PROTEIN	FAT
8g	4g	3g	7g

Buttered Cabbage Ribbons

This is a really good alternative to ribbons of pasta such as pappardelle or tagliolini. White cabbage is firmer and will take a couple of minutes longer to cook to transform into soft, tender ribbons; it is the perfect foil for a rich ragù. Savoy cabbage is bright green and pretty when cooked; it is excellent with pasta sauces.

1. To make the cabbage ribbons, cut the cabbage in half and remove the hard core and outer raggedy leaves. Lay the two halves, flat-side down, on a chopping board and use a sharp knife to slice it into 1.5cm- (⅝ inch)-wide ribbons.

2. Put the cabbage, butter, 3 tablespoons of water and some seasoning in the drawer or a silicone liner and air fry at 200°C (400°F) for 5 minutes for soft cabbage such as sweetheart and up to 7 minutes for thicker cabbage such as kale ribbons, stirring twice during the cooking time.

3. Drain the cabbage in a sieve and tip into a warm bowl. Dress with a sauce of your choice and enjoy!

200g (7oz) cabbage ribbons
10g (¼oz) butter
salt and pepper

Per serving: 61kcal			
NET CARBS	FIBRE	PROTEIN	FAT
4g	2g	1g	4g

Peas, Lettuce and Spring Onions

Serves 2

This is one of my favourite French vegetable dishes. Soft lettuce, sweet peas and oniony butter: 'Délicieuse'. Serve this with the Pork Steaks with Sage and Garlic (see page 117) and you'll think you're in a Parisian bistro.

1. Put all the ingredients, with the cut side of the lettuce facing downward, into the base of the drawer. Air fry at 180°C (350°F) for 10 minutes, turning the lettuces over to expose the cut side halfway through.

2. Tip the vegetables on to a warm plate or bowl to serve with the buttery juices.

100g (3½oz) frozen peas
15g (½oz) butter
2 spring onions, roughly chopped
2 little gem lettuces, halved lengthways, or 1 romaine heart, quartered lengthways
salt and pepper

Per serving: 107kcal			
NET CARBS	**FIBRE**	**PROTEIN**	**FAT**
6g	5g	4g	7g

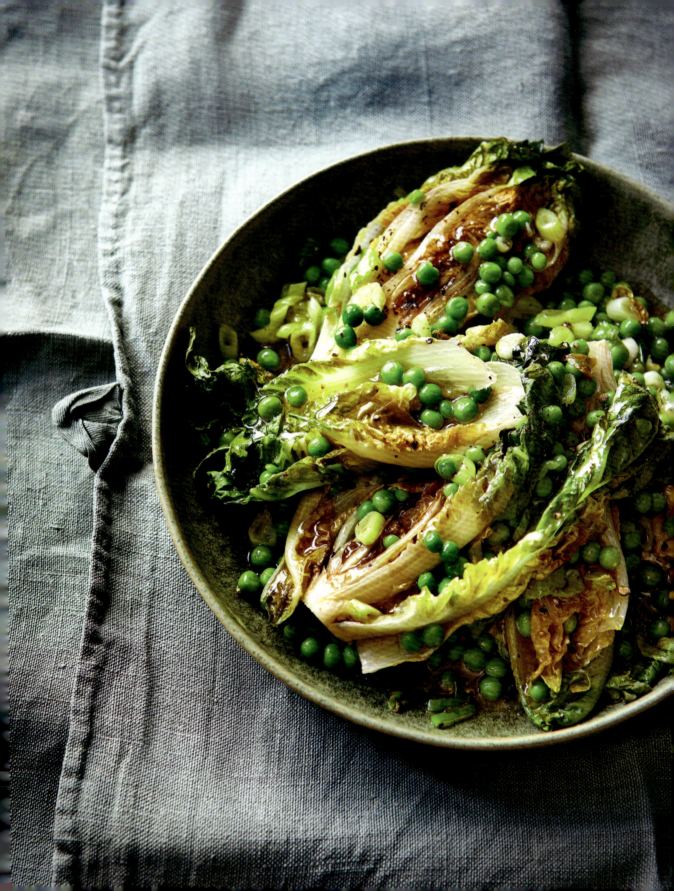

Sautéed Mushrooms

This has to be one of my favourite air fryer recipes. I love garlicky mushrooms, but they always stick to the frying pan unless I use copious amounts of oil. Now I can air fry them in 8 minutes and they are beautifully tender and juicy. Have them as part of breakfast with eggs or bacon or try them on toasted Low-carb Bread (see page 156) topped with a couple of fried eggs.

1. Put the mushrooms into the drawer or a silicone liner and spray or drizzle with the oil as you toss them around with a spatula. Add some salt and plenty of pepper, along with the garlic, butter and herbs and toss them again.

2. Air fry at 200°C (400°F) for 8 minutes, moving and tossing them once halfway through. The mushrooms are done when they are just soft and lightly browned.

3. Serve straight away or keep warm until you need them.

300g (10½oz) mushrooms, trimmed and sliced
1 tablespoon extra-virgin olive oil
1 garlic clove, peeled and lightly crushed using the flat of a knife
1 tablespoon butter
1 rosemary or thyme sprig (optional)
salt and pepper

Per serving: 143kcal			
NET CARBS	FIBRE	PROTEIN	FAT
3g	2g	5g	13g

The Diabetes Air Fryer Cookbook

Creamy Spinach with Nutmeg

Frozen spinach has all the nutrients of fresh, so don't disregard it. This is the French way to eat spinach and it is utterly delicious! With this recipe, the spinach can go from freezer to table in less than 20 minutes! I could eat a whole plate of these greens for breakfast, lunch or dinner, as a side or with a poached egg on top.

I'm a bit of a forager, so I'll add in edible weeds from my garden such as wild rocket, ground elder, nettle and dandelion leaves, adding fibre and a diversity of vitamins and minerals. Steam or boil them briefly first and then drain, as loose dry leaves can float upward toward the element.

Defrosting frozen spinach in the air fryer gets rid of the water: two jobs in one. I love it!

1. Defrost the spinach on the base of the drawer at 180°C (350°F) for 10 minutes, turning it twice during this time. Remove the drawer and pour away any water. Usually, I find the water has evaporated and this isn't necessary.

2. Add the butter, cream, nutmeg and seasoning and stir through. Put the drawer back in the air fryer and cook at 200°C (400°F) for another 4 minutes. Taste and adjust the seasoning as necessary.

400g (14oz) frozen spinach
15g (½oz) salted butter
4 tablespoons double cream
¼ teaspoon ground nutmeg
salt and pepper

Tips and tricks
Fresh baby spinach should be washed and dressed with oil and seasoning (weighing it down so it doesn't blow around), then it can be cooked as above in the drawer for 5 minutes.

Per serving: 195kcal			
NET CARBS	FIBRE	PROTEIN	FAT
3g	8g	16g	7g

Crispy Broccoli and Cauliflower

Crispy florets of broccoli or cauliflower in 10 minutes! Now there is no excuse not to eat your greens.

1. Toss the broccoli thoroughly with the oil, seasoning and/or any additional flavourings in a bowl. Put the florets in a single layer on a crisper in the drawer without overcrowding them.

2. Air fry at 170°C (340°F) for 5–7 minutes, or until the broccoli is crisp around the edges and the stalks are tender. Check after 5 minutes and give the drawer a shake. (I don't always turn the florets halfway through if the air is circulating through the crisper.)

3. Serve warm.

150g (5½oz) broccoli and/or cauliflower, tough, large stalks removed (reserve for another dish), cut into 4cm (1½ inch) florets
1 tablespoon extra-virgin olive oil
salt or tamari (optional)

Additional flavourings (optional)
1 teaspoon grated garlic or granules
1 teaspoon spice mix (such as curry powder, chaat masala, smoked paprika)
1 tablespoon finely grated Parmesan, Grana Padano or vegetarian Italian-style hard cheese

Per serving: 85kcal			
NET CARBS	FIBRE	PROTEIN	FAT
3g	2g	2g	7g
Per serving with Parmesan: 90kcal			
NET CARBS	FIBRE	PROTEIN	FAT
3g	2g	3g	8g

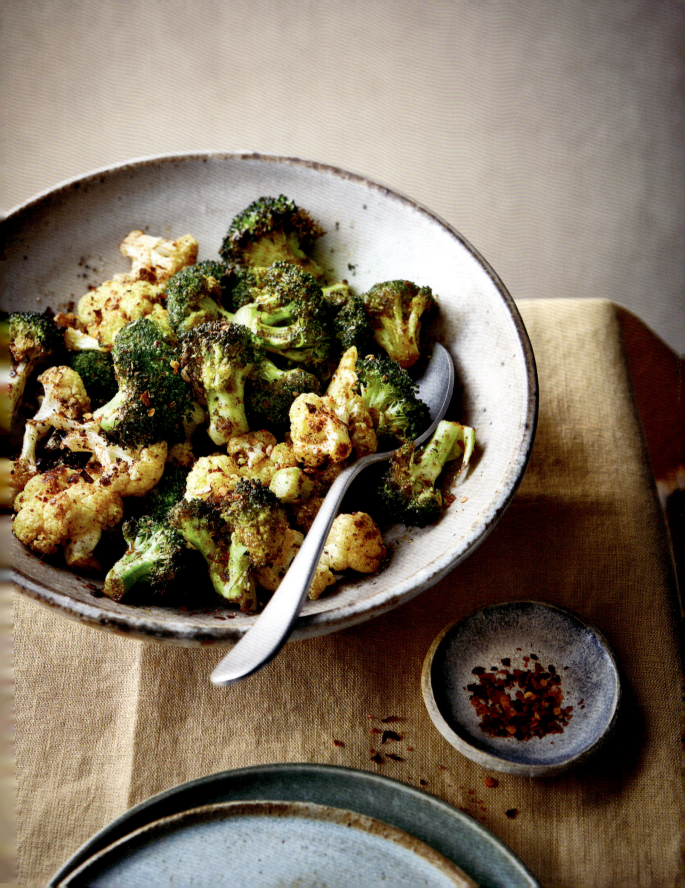

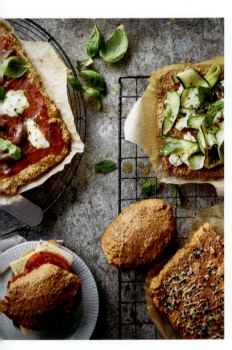
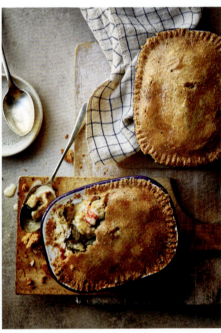
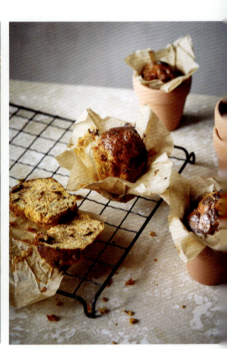

BAKES

Low-carb Bread (pictured on pages 160–1)

Bread, beautiful bread! We all love it, but unfortunately it can be responsible for a huge rise in blood glucose. I know from wearing a continuous glucose monitor in my arm that measures my glucose response, that even the most gorgeous, artisan sourdough gives me a peak of energy followed by a trough of tiredness. The oh-so-useful, everyday sandwich is really not ideal if you have type 2 diabetes.

However, I have been determined to find a solution so that once more those watching their glucose levels can enjoy the comfort and ease of a humble bread roll. This is my best recipe yet and tastes like Irish soda bread. These rolls are quick to make, last for 4 days in the refrigerator and freeze well for up to 3 months.

Depending on the size of your air fryer, you may be able to make 2 or 4 rolls at the same time. You can also cook the mixture in containers such as lined ramekins or even terracotta flowerpots. I like to carefully cut mine in half horizontally with a serrated knife so that I can fill a buttered roll with bacon, fried eggs or a tasty sandwich filling or even toast them and enjoy with soup. I usually use wheat bran, the husk of the wheat kernel, to give texture and flavour, but if you are looking for something gluten-free, see the oat bran version opposite. Wheat bran does vary, if you have the heavier, finely ground version, you may find 3 tablespoons isn't enough to bind the dough, so add up to 2 tablespoons more.

Nut-free? If you can't eat nuts, grind linseed, sunflower or other mixed seeds to a flour in a small food processor and substitute them for the ground almonds in the recipes.

1 quantity of dough (see opposite)

1. Put a piece of nonstick baking paper cut to the size of the drawer on a crisper or the base of the air fryer. It needs to be just big enough to be under the rolls but not big enough to flap about.

2. Use a spoon to transfer the dough to the drawer in 2 mounds. Using the back of the spoon, spread the mixture to make 2 flattened ovals, each around 12 x 8cm (4½ x 3¼ inches) and about 2cm (¾ inch) thick. If you prefer and your air fryer allows the space, do make circles of different measures instead.

3. Air fry at 200°C (400°F) for 8 minutes, or until solid to the touch and lightly browned. Remove from the paper and eat straight away, or cool and store in the refrigerator in an airtight container for up to 3 days or in the freezer for up to 3 months. I slice the rolls in half before freezing and toast them to defrost.

Low-carb Wheat Bran Dough

1. Mix all the ingredients together in a small bowl until blended. Leave it for 5 minutes to absorb the liquid. If your eggs are large and the mixture is still very wet, then add a little more bran to thicken it. At this point it can be made into rolls, pizza or flatbread.

Tips and tricks

Flowerpot bread rolls: Line 2 small terracotta flowerpots around 6cm (2½ inches) across, 7cm (2¾ inches) deep with wetted and scrunched nonstick baking paper. Put the mixture in the pots and bake at 180°C (350°F) for 10 minutes.

Rosemary and Cheddar: Flavour either of the Low-carb Dough recipes with 1 teaspoon of finely chopped rosemary and 15g (½oz) finely grated hard cheese such as Cheddar or Parmesan, Grana Padano or vegetarian Italian-style hard cheese.

Makes 2 bread rolls, 1 pizza to serve 2 or 1 flatbread to serve 4

2 eggs
50g (1¾oz) ground almonds
¼ teaspoon salt
3 tablespoons (10g/¼oz) coarse wheat bran (see introduction opposite), plus extra as necessary
¼ teaspoon baking powder

Per serving of rosemary and Cheddar: 15kcal			
NET CARBS	FIBRE	PROTEIN	FAT
0.5g	0g	1g	1g

Gluten-free Low-carb Oat Bran Dough

Try to find an oat bran that has plenty of coarse husks in it. Brands vary and one with more husk contains around 50g carbs per 100g (3½oz), while others contain more oats and are finely ground; they can contain 60g carbs per 100g (3½oz). Ground linseed has one-quarter of the carbs compared to oat bran but has less flavour, so for a savoury bread I would add 15g (½oz) grated hard cheese such as Parmesan, Grana Padano or vegetarian Italian-style hard cheese, it will only add a tiny amount of carbs but gives more taste.

1. Mix all the ingredients together in a small bowl until blended. Leave it for 10 minutes to absorb the liquid. If it is still very wet, add a little more bran or linseed to thicken it. At this point, it can be made into rolls, pizza or flatbread.

Makes 2 bread rolls, 1 pizza to serve 2 or 1 flatbread to serve 4

2 eggs
40g (1½oz) ground almonds
good pinch of salt
25g (1oz) gluten-free oat bran or ground linseed
½ teaspoon baking powder

Per roll or flowerpot bread with wheat bran dough: 205kcal			
NET CARBS	FIBRE	PROTEIN	FAT
4g	4g	10g	16g
Per slice of flatbread with wheat bran dough: 102kcal			
NET CARBS	FIBRE	PROTEIN	FAT
2g	2g	5g	8g

Per roll or flowerpot bread with oat bran dough: 240kcal			
NET CARBS	FIBRE	PROTEIN	FAT
8g	3g	12g	17g
Per slice of flatbread with oat bran dough: 120kcal			
NET CARBS	FIBRE	PROTEIN	FAT
4g	2g	6g	9g

Per roll or flowerpot bread with linseed dough: 261kcal			
NET CARBS	FIBRE	PROTEIN	FAT
2g	5g	12g	21g
Per slice of flatbread with linseed dough: 130kcal			
NET CARBS	FIBRE	PROTEIN	FAT
1g	2g	6g	11g

Low-carb Flatbreads and Pizza
(pictured overleaf)

Pizza is loved the world over, as it is one of the most umami-rich
(savoury and tasty) foods we can find. However, it is high in carbs –
from the base to the tomato sauce – and with the fat from the cheese
is usually highly calorific, so pizza shouldn't be an everyday food.

My low-carb pizza, with all the nutrition it contains, will see you
through to the next meal without wanting a snack or having the
highs and lows of glucose spikes. The base can be cooled, covered
and kept in the refrigerator for up to 3 days or frozen for up to
3 months. Defrost before use. I use inexpensive cows' milk
mozzarella for this.

1. Trim a paper baking liner so that the edges are only 3cm
   (1¼ inches) high, otherwise it will flap down into the bread.
   Put it in the drawer and give it a few sprays with oil.

2. Spoon the dough on to the liner in the drawer. Use the back of the
   spoon to spread it out to around 2cm (¾ inch) thick. Bake at 200°C
   (400°F) for 7 minutes, or until golden brown and firm to the touch.
   Remove the bread and liner from the drawer and put the bread
   upside down on a chopping board to cool. Reserve the liner.

3. Meanwhile, mix all the tomato sauce ingredients together in
   a small bowl, seasoning with the salt to taste.

4. To complete the pizza, put the base back on the paper liner,
   top-side up. Leaving a finger-width border around the edge, spoon
   over the tomato sauce in an even layer. Add the mozzarella and
   olives and then put the pizza into the drawer on the liner. Air fry
   at 200°C (400°F) for 5 minutes, or until the cheese is bubbling
   and the crust is crisp and browned.

5. Remove using an angled slice, then serve with the basil leaves and
   a good grind of pepper.

For the dough
extra-virgin olive oil
1 quantity of Low-carb Wheat Bran
   Dough or Gluten-free Low-carb
   Oat Bran Dough (see page 157)

For the tomato sauce
4 tablespoons tomato passata
   (sieved tomatoes) or mashed
   canned Italian tomatoes
1 teaspoon dried oregano
¼–½ teaspoon salt

For the topping
60g (2¼oz) mozzarella cheese,
   torn into pieces
25g (1oz) black olives, pitted
a small handful of basil leaves,
   to serve
freshly ground black pepper

Per serving with wheat bran dough: 324kcal			
NET CARBS	FIBRE	PROTEIN	FAT
6g	5g	17g	24g
Per pizza with oat bran dough: 379kcal			
NET CARBS	FIBRE	PROTEIN	FAT
5g	5g	19g	30g

Feta, Courgette and Mint Flatbread
(pictured overleaf)

Serves 4

Enjoy this flatbread cut into squares for sharing, or use it to add protein and satiety to a simple salad or packed lunch. To contain and cook the flatbread, you will need a liner made of nonstick baking paper or silicone.

extra-virgin olive oil
1 quantity of Low-carb Wheat Bran
   Dough or Gluten-free Low-carb
   Oat Bran Dough (see page 157)
1 courgette, thinly sliced using a
   vegetable peeler or sharp knife
75g (2½oz) feta cheese
handful of mint leaves, torn
salt and pepper

1. Trim a baking paper liner so that the edges are only 3cm (1¼ inches) high, otherwise it will flap down into the bread. Put it in the drawer and give it a few sprays with oil.

2. Spoon the dough on to the liner in the drawer. Use the back of the spoon to spread it out to around 2cm (¾ inch) thick and bake at 200°C (400°F) for 6–9 minutes, or until golden brown and firm to the touch. Remove the bread and liner from the drawer, peel off the paper liner, then put the bread on a chopping board.

3. Meanwhile, put the courgette in a bowl and spray it with oil. Season with salt and pepper and toss through. Put it into a drawer if you have a spare one (or use the one from the flatbread) and air fry at 200°C (400°F) for 6–7 minutes, or until lightly browned in places and just softened. Leave in the drawer if you have 2 or tip out on to a plate.

4. Spray or brush a crisper with oil and put it into the drawer. Put the bread on top and crumble over the feta cheese, then give it a couple of sprays of oil. Put the bread back into the air fryer and cook at 200°C (400°F) for 3–5 minutes, or until the cheese has just softened.

5. Remove the bread using an angled slice. On top, pile the courgette ribbons, add the mint leaves, spray some oil and grind plenty of pepper. Cut into slices and serve straight away.

Tips and tricks

Sautéed mushroom, goats' cheese and thyme flatbread:
Instead of the courgette, use half the quantity of Sautéed Mushrooms on page 150 (making sure they are quite dry after cooking). Replace the feta with crumbly goats' cheese and the mint with thyme leaves.

Garlic naan (pictured overleaf):
When the flatbread is cooked, spread the top with 15g (½oz) soft butter mixed with 5g (⅛oz) minced garlic (or frozen or granules), ½ teaspoon of black onion (nigella) seeds and a pinch of salt and return to the air fryer at 200°C (400°F) for 3 minutes, or until melted.

Per slice with wheat bran dough: 190kcal			
NET CARBS	FIBRE	PROTEIN	FAT
3g	3g	8g	15g
Per slice with oat bran dough: 201kcal			
NET CARBS	FIBRE	PROTEIN	FAT
6g	3g	9g	16g

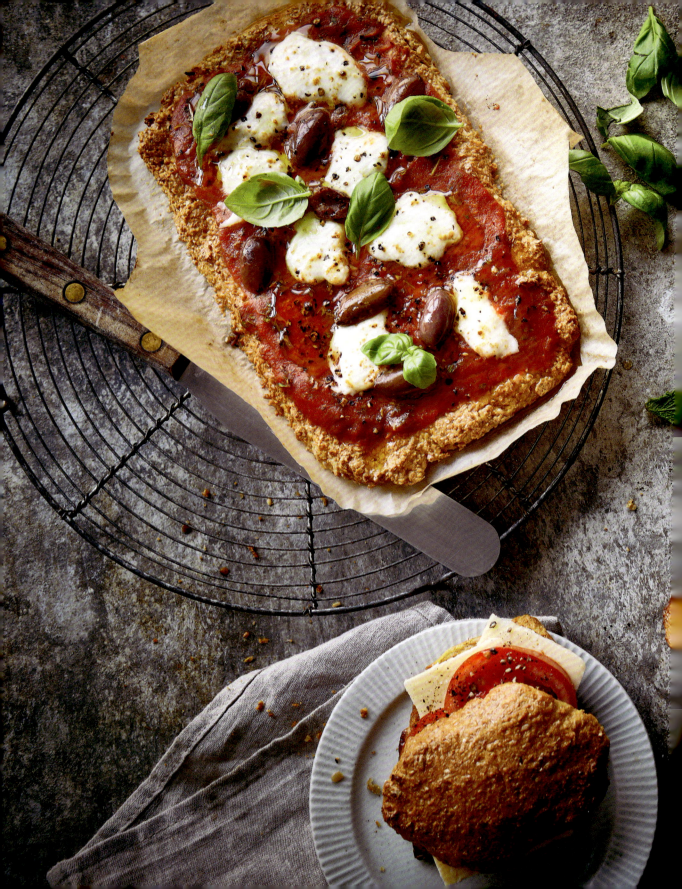

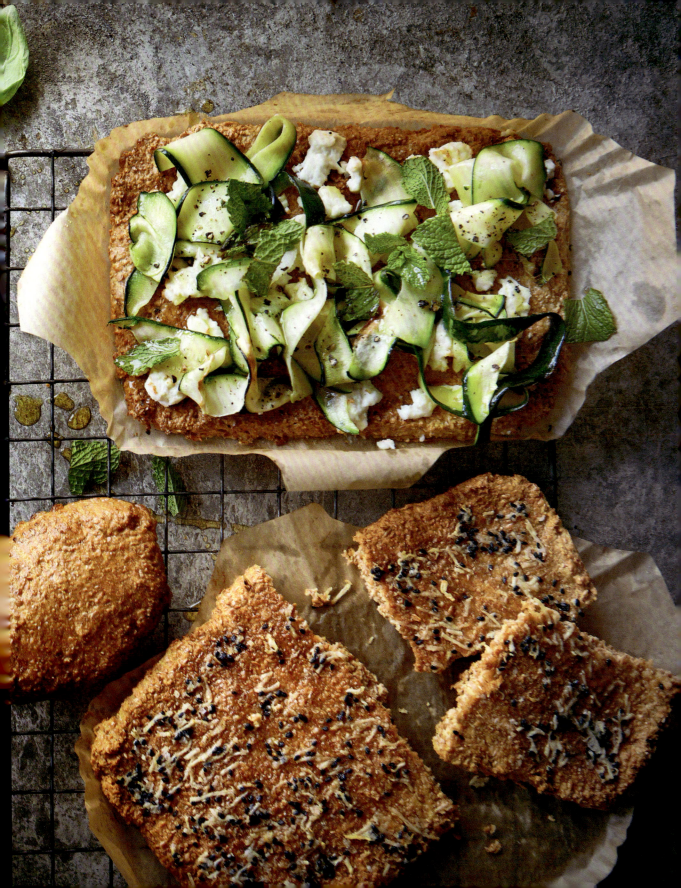

Mixed Seed and Walnut Loaf

Makes 1 loaf
(16 slices)

I was thrilled to be able to cook a loaf of this bread in my air fryer. No more heating up the whole oven any more. This bread can be sliced, wrapped and frozen for up to 3 months, then toasted from frozen, or it keeps in the refrigerator for up to 5 days. If you don't have a suitable loaf tin, use any small-sized ovenproof dish and line it with nonstick baking paper.

1. Spray a 450g (1lb) loaf tin (making sure it fits in your air fryer) with some oil.

2. Use a metal spoon to mix all the dry ingredients together in a large mixing bowl. Vigorously stir in the mozzarella, 5 tablespoons of cold water and the eggs. When you have a well-combined dough, use your hands to gather it into a ball and remove it from the bowl. Shape the dough between your hands and put it into the prepared loaf tin. Spray the top of the loaf with oil and put a piece of tin foil over the loaf, tucking it under the tin so that it can't fly away in the fan.

3. Bake the loaf at 160°C (325°F) for 30 minutes. Remove the tin foil and bake for a further 30 minutes, or until lightly browned and firm to the touch.

4. Remove from the air fryer, turn the loaf out of the tin and leave to cool on a wire rack before slicing to serve.

Tips and tricks
Add 2 teaspoons of caraway seeds to the dough to give it the flavour of rye bread.

extra-virgin olive oil
100g (3½oz) mixed seeds (such as pumpkin, flax, sunflower, sesame)
100g (3½oz) ground almonds
75g (2½oz) walnuts, roughly chopped
10g (¼oz) wheat bran
1 teaspoon baking powder
½ teaspoon salt
100g (3½oz) mozzarella cheese, coarsely grated
3 eggs, beaten

Per slice: 136kcal			
NET CARBS	FIBRE	PROTEIN	FAT
2g	2g	6g	12g

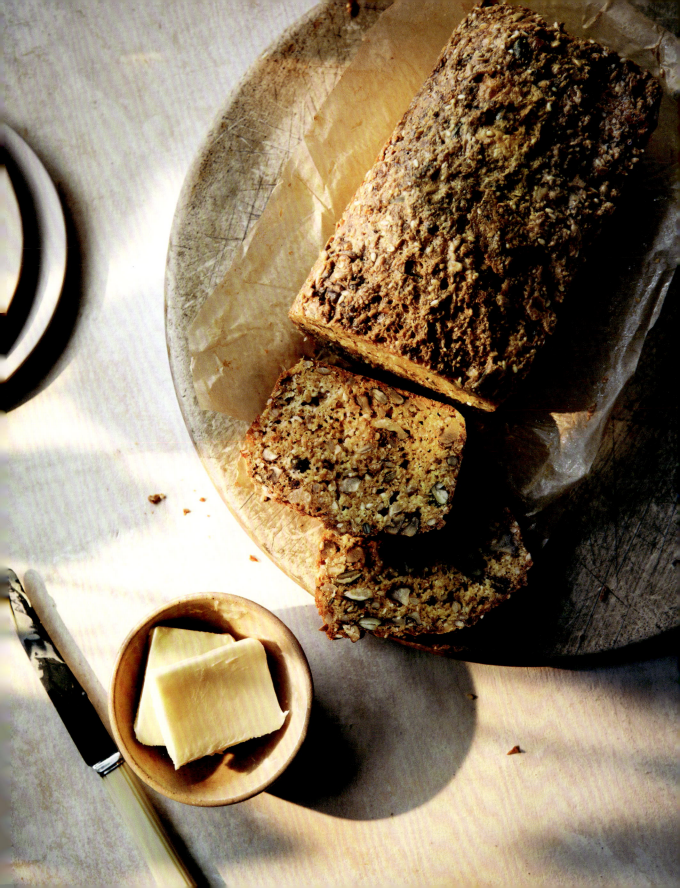

Sausage Rolls

These crunchy bites are good for a light lunch with soup or to take on your travels. Unlike traditional pastry sausage rolls, these won't give you such a spike of blood glucose. Do seek out good-quality sausages with no or little added rusk and a high meat content. I use inexpensive cows' milk mozzarella for this rather than expensive buffalo milk; it comes in 200g (7oz) logs.

1. Cut 2 pieces of nonstick baking paper to roughly 40 x 30cm (16 x 12 inches).

2. To make the pastry, use a food processor to blend all the ingredients together; or coarsely grate the mozzarella, put it into a bowl with the remaining ingredients and then use a spoon to stir and squeeze them together to form a smooth, thick dough.

3. Using your hands, gather the dough into a ball and place it on a piece of the baking paper. Lay the other piece of baking paper on top and use a rolling pin to roll the dough into a rectangle about 36 x 22cm (14 x 8½ inches) and 3mm (⅛ inch) thick. You can cut away misshapen pieces and add them back in as necessary to make your rectangle. You shouldn't have any leftover dough.

4. Score a line down the sausages and peel away the skin. Leaving a 3cm (1¼ inch) border, lay 2 sausages, side by side, along the short edge of the rectangle. Obviously, some sausages are shorter or fatter than others, so squeeze or stretch the sausagemeat accordingly to fit the length. Use the baking paper to lift the pastry from each edge and roll up to cover the sausages. Press the pastry layers together to form a seal (of around 5mm/¼ inch), cut the pastry and slide the roll to one side. Repeat with the next 2 sausages and so on until the sausages and dough are used up.

5. Use a serrated knife to gently cut each roll into 6 pieces, cleaning the knife frequently, so it doesn't stick and tear the pastry.

6. Spray or brush a crisper with oil, place it in the drawer and then carefully place the sausage rolls on it. Brush with the egg yolk and bake at 160°C (325°F) for 15 minutes, or until the pastry is golden brown. You may need to cook them in batches. Check the sausage is cooked by cutting the largest roll in half and making sure it is no longer pink in the middle.

7. Serve the sausage rolls warm or at room temperature. Once cooled, they will keep in a sealed container in the refrigerator for up to 3 days or in the freezer for up to 3 months.

6 high-meat-content, gluten-free sausages (approx. 400g/14oz)
extra-virgin olive oil
1 egg yolk, beaten, to glaze

For the pastry
175g (6oz) ground almonds
200g (7oz) mozzarella cheese
25g (1oz) wheat bran or oat bran
½ teaspoon salt

Per sausage roll: 125kcal			
NET CARBS	FIBRE	PROTEIN	FAT
2g	2g	6g	10g

Veggie Roll Filling

1. Whizz the oats in a food processor until they resemble sand. Mix the oats together with the remaining ingredients in a large bowl, using a large spatula, adding a little salt to taste, until well blended.

2. Divide the mixture into 3, then lightly wet your hands and roll each section of the mixture into a sausage shape. Use this instead of the sausages to fill the sausage rolls, following the recipe opposite. Once cooled, they will keep in a sealed container in the refrigerator for up to 3 days or in the freezer for up to 3 months.

50g (1¾oz) rolled oats
150g (5½oz) cooked beetroot, coarsely grated
100g (3½oz) feta cheese, coarsely grated
1 teaspoon roughly chopped thyme leaves
1 large egg
1 heaped teaspoon ground cumin
salt

Per veggie roll: 141kcal			
NET CARBS	FIBRE	PROTEIN	FAT
4g	3g	5g	11g

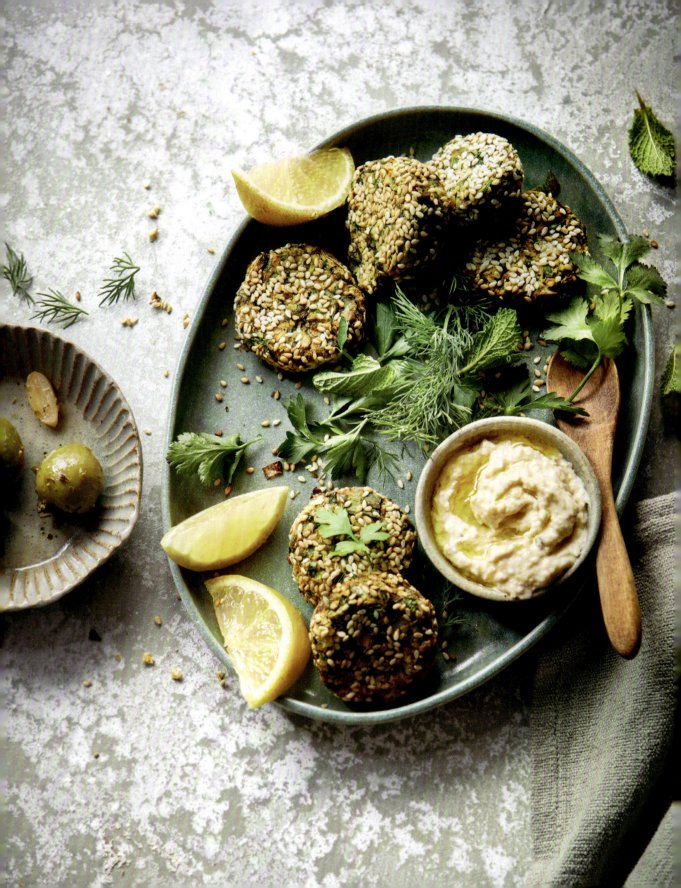

Falafel

**Makes approx. 16 falafel
(serves 4)**

Crunchy falafel are a great choice when catering for vegans and
vegetarians, but can be high in carbs and low in protein. In this
recipe, the carbs are lowered by using spinach, fewer chickpeas
and no flour. I use frozen spinach to make these; it doesn't need to
be cooked, but do make sure it is defrosted and squeezed very dry
before using.

Falafel mixture is usually rested for 30 minutes before cooking,
but I haven't found that necessary with this recipe. However, if
you want to prepare it in advance, it will be fine, covered, in the
refrigerator for up to a day and can be cooked when you are ready.
Serve with Hummus, Spicy Roasted Tomato Salsa or Guacamole
(see pages 194, 91 and 194) and salad.

1. Thoroughly spray or brush a crisper in the drawer with oil.

2. Put the seeds on a large plate. Dry the chickpeas between 2 pieces
   of kitchen paper or a clean tea towel.

3. Put the chickpeas, along with all the remaining ingredients and
   a generous amount of pepper, into a food processor and pulse
   the mixture to a rough paste. If you don't have a food processor,
   mash the chickpeas with a potato masher, then add the rest of the
   ingredients. Mash again until well combined. Taste the mixture and
   add more spices or salt as necessary.

4. Roll the mixture into 16 walnut-sized balls (around 25g/1oz each)
   in your hands and flatten gently into circles around 5cm (2 inches)
   across and 1.5cm (⅝ inch) thick. Press the shaped falafels into the
   seeds to coat them.

5. Lay them on the oiled crisper (you may have to do this in batches)
   and air fry at 200°C (400°F) for 12–15 minutes, or until firm and
   lightly browned.

6. Serve warm, or at room temperature, with lemon wedges.

extra-virgin olive oil
50g (1¾oz) sesame seeds
400g (14oz) can chickpeas, well
    drained
1 small onion or 120g (4¼oz) spring
    onions, roughly chopped
1 fat garlic clove, roughly chopped
25g (1oz) fresh soft herbs (such as
    coriander or parsley), stalks and
    leaves
100g (3½oz) very well-squeezed
    cooked spinach (300g/10½oz
    frozen weight)
1 teaspoon ground cumin, or more
    to taste
1 teaspoon sweet paprika, or more
    to taste
½ teaspoon salt, or more to taste
freshly ground black pepper
lemon wedges, to serve

Per falafel: 45kcal			
NET CARBS	FIBRE	PROTEIN	FAT
3g	1g	2g	2g

Italian Chicken, Vegetable and Cheese Pies

In Italian this would be called *torte salate*, savoury pies. I love the cheesy, creamy filling around roast vegetables and chicken, but you could use leftover cooked ham or pork instead or skip the meat and go veggie. I've given a list of low-carb vegetables to use, as when I'm making these, I use up what's in my refrigerator, but you could use just one or two types. Make four small or two large pies according to the size of your air fryer and the containers that will fit inside. The uncooked pies can be chilled and frozen for another day (see tip). Once cooked, the pies will reheat in air fryer at 160°C (325°F) for 10 minutes. Enjoy the pies on their own or with a side salad.

1. Put the vegetables, garlic, herbs and seasoning into the drawer without a crisper or into an ovenproof dish. Spray or drizzle with the oil and toss through. Air fry at 200°C (400°F) for 10–12 minutes until just cooked through, tossing a couple of times.

2. Remove the vegetables with a slotted spoon and set aside in a bowl, leaving any oil in the drawer. Discard the sprigs.

3. Put the chicken into the drawer with a little more salt and pepper and give it a good shake. Air fry the chicken at 200°C (400°F) for 8–10 minutes until cooked through. Check it is done by cutting the biggest piece in half and making sure there are no pink juices running from it.

4. Remove the chicken with a slotted spoon and add it to the vegetables. Pour any juices into a small bowl.

5. Beat the eggs in a mixing bowl and spoon 1 tablespoon into a small bowl for brushing the pies. Set aside. To the rest, add the crème fraîche, Parmesan and a couple of tablespoons of any juices left from cooking the meat (if there aren't any, don't worry). Season with a pinch of salt and pepper.

6. Toss the vegetables and chicken together in the bowl and then distribute the mixture between 2 medium or 4 small pie dishes. Pour the cheesy cream evenly over the vegetables.

Continued over page

For the filling
1kg (2lb 4oz) low-carb vegetables such as onion, leek, spring onion, courgette, aubergine, broccoli, cauliflower or mushrooms, chopped into 2cm (¾ inch) dice
2 garlic cloves, roughly chopped
2 rosemary or thyme sprigs or 1 teaspoon dried Italian herbs
2 tablespoons extra-virgin olive oil
300g (10½oz) boneless, skinless chicken thighs, cut into bite-sized chunks
2 eggs
100ml (3½fl oz) crème fraîche or double cream
25g (1oz) Parmesan, Grana Padano or Italian-style hard cheese, finely grated
salt and pepper

For the pastry
100g (3½oz) mozzarella cheese
75g (2½oz) ground almonds
15g (½oz) wheat bran or coarse oat bran
¼ teaspoon salt

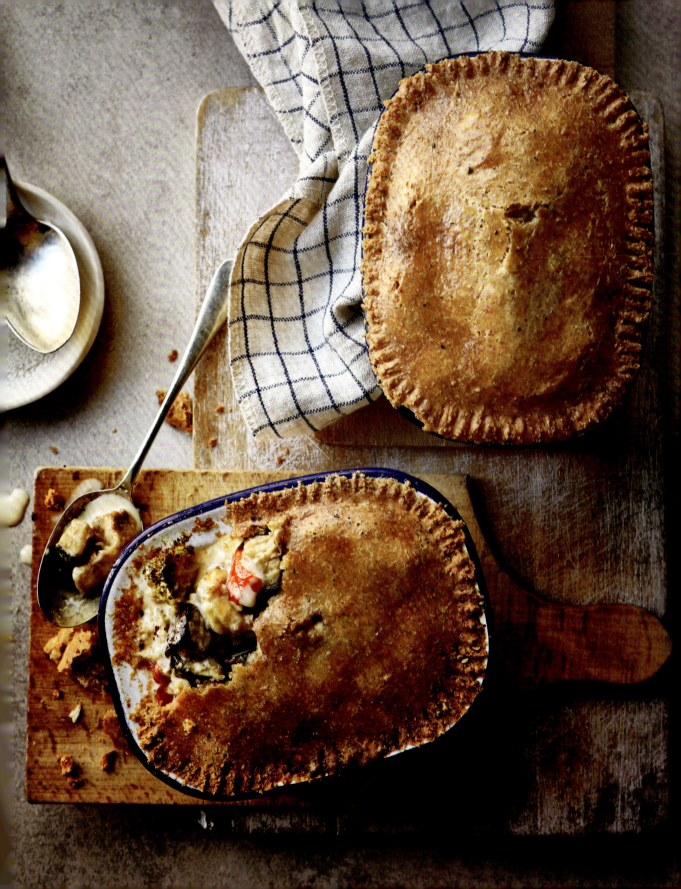

Italian Chicken, Vegetable and Cheese Pies (continued)

7. To make the pastry, use a food processor to blend all the ingredients together to make a smooth paste. To do this by hand, coarsely grate the mozzarella into a bowl, add the rest of the ingredients and use a spoon to stir and squeeze them together to form a smooth, thick dough. Use a spatula to remove the mixture, or use your hands to gather it into a ball, and put the dough on a piece of nonstick baking paper.

8. Lay another piece of nonstick baking paper on top and use a rolling pin to roll the dough to 5mm (¼ inch) thick. Cut the dough into 2 or 4 equal pieces to cover the pies. You can cut, gather and re-roll the pastry between the paper as necessary to make your pastry lids. Using a fork, fix the pastry to each dish by pressing it down all along the edge, and then trim off any edges.

9. Brush the reserved beaten egg over the pies.

10. Make a small hole in the centre of each pie to allow the steam to escape. Bake in the air fryer at 160°C (325°F) for 17–20 minutes, or until golden brown. Serve hot.

Tips and tricks

Cool the filling to room temperature before filling the pie dishes. Add the pastry, don't brush them with the egg and freeze them, uncovered, for 1–2 hours until firm. Wrap in nonstick baking paper and put into a container. Return to the freezer for up to 3 months. Defrost before cooking.

Per serving with wheat bran: 572kcal			
NET CARBS	FIBRE	PROTEIN	FAT
11g	7g	31g	44g
Per serving with oat bran: 574kcal			
NET CARBS	FIBRE	PROTEIN	FAT
13g	5g	31g	44g

The Diabetes Air Fryer Cookbook

Savoury Feta and Black Onion Seed Muffins

These are great to take to work; enjoy them warm (reheated in a microwave or air fryer) or at room temperature for breakfast or lunch, either on their own or with cream cheese and tomatoes.

1. Mix all the ingredients, apart from the feta, together in a mixing bowl, adding some salt and pepper. When well blended, gently stir in the feta so that the crumbled lumps remain.

2. Transfer the mixture into 4 silicone muffin moulds, 7cm (2¾ inches) in diameter and 3.5cm (1¼ inches) deep. Place in the drawer and air fry at 180°C (350°F) for 11–12 minutes, or until a skewer poked into the middle comes out clean; if it is wet, put them back into the air fryer for another few minutes.

3. Serve warm with cream cheese and tomatoes or leave to cool on a wire rack and take to work. The muffins can be stored an airtight container in in the refrigerator for up to 3 days or frozen for up to 3 months.

4 eggs
200g (7oz) ground almonds
200g (7oz) courgette, coarsely grated
1 teaspoon baking powder
1 teaspoon salt
1 teaspoon dried oregano
2 teaspoons black onion (nigella) seeds
1 hot red chilli, finely chopped, or ¼ teaspoon chilli flakes
50g (1¾oz) feta, crumbled
salt and pepper

Per muffin: 426kcal			
NET CARBS	FIBRE	PROTEIN	FAT
5g	4g	19g	38g

Banana and Chocolate Muffins

Ideally serve these warm straight from the air fryer while the chocolate is still molten. A couple of these are perfect for breakfast on the go, or you could add one to a packed lunch. Serve with a dollop of cream cheese or Greek yogurt and berries. Choosing the 'bake' setting on an air fryer often means the fan will be less strong, which helps when you are cooking anything that needs to cook through rather than burn on top.

I love these baked in my mini terracotta flowerpots, which are approx. 6cm (2½ inches) across and 6cm (2½ inches) deep. I line them with scrunched and wetted nonstick baking paper, but the muffins will work equally well in 7cm- (2¾ inch)-diameter, 3.5cm- (1½ inch)-deep silicone muffin moulds.

1. Mash the banana with a fork in a mixing bowl. Stir in the rest of the ingredients until thoroughly combined. Distribute the mixture evenly between 4 lined mini flowerpots or 6 silicone muffin moulds.

2. Bake in the air fryer at 160°C (325°F) for 12–15 minutes, or until firm and cooked through.

3. The smaller ones can be turned out straight away on to a wire rack, but leave the flowerpot muffins for 10 minutes to cool before turning out. Serve warm.

1 small banana (approx. 120g/4¼oz)
2 eggs
1 teaspoon vanilla extract
60g (2¼oz) ground almonds
50g (1¾oz) chopped walnuts
½ teaspoon baking powder
15g (½oz) dark chocolate (at least 85% cocoa solids), chopped

Tips and tricks

Raspberry and banana seeded muffins: Instead of the chocolate and walnuts, mix in 75g (2½oz) raspberries and 50g (1¾oz) mixed seeds. Mix and bake as above.

These are completely lovely while warm with a cup of coffee. No one would know there is no sugar in the recipe as the banana and raspberry have enough natural sweetness.

Nut-free muffins: For nut-free muffins, use a small processor to grind the same amount of sunflower or mixed seeds to a fine powder and use this instead of the ground almonds, and omit the chopped walnuts. Mix and bake as above

Per banana and chocolate flowerpot muffin: 243kcal			
NET CARBS	FIBRE	PROTEIN	FAT
8g	3g	9g	20g
Per small muffin: 161kcal			
NET CARBS	FIBRE	PROTEIN	FAT
6g	2g	6g	13g

Per raspberry and banana seeded flowerpot muffin: 222kcal			
NET CARBS	FIBRE	PROTEIN	FAT
9g	5g	9g	16g
Per small muffin: 148kcal			
NET CARBS	FIBRE	PROTEIN	FAT
6g	3g	6g	11g

Per nut-free flowerpot muffin: 224kcal			
NET CARBS	FIBRE	PROTEIN	FAT
9g	4g	9g	17g
Per small muffin: 149kcal			
NET CARBS	FIBRE	PROTEIN	FAT
6g	3g	6g	11g

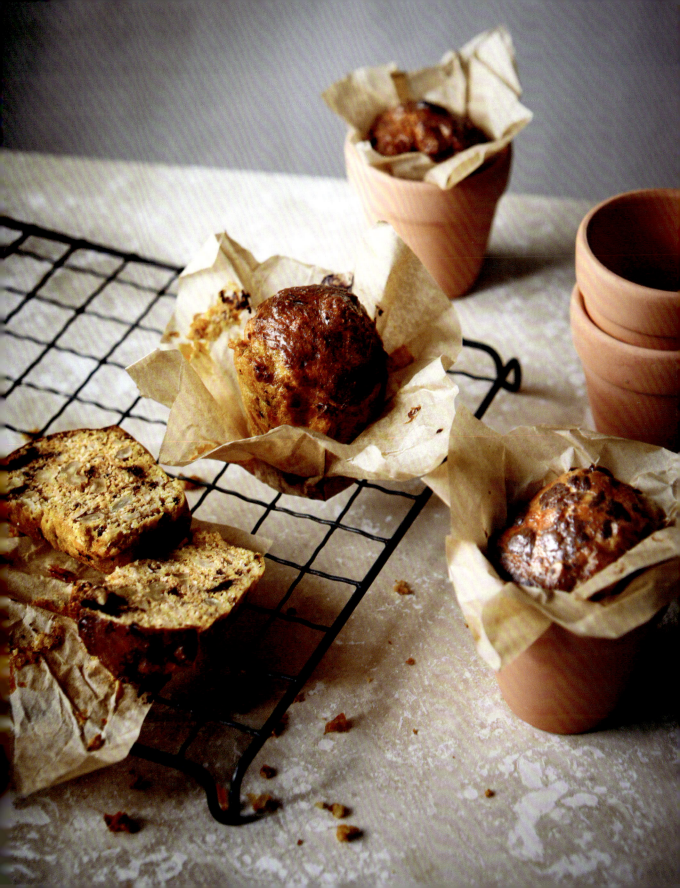

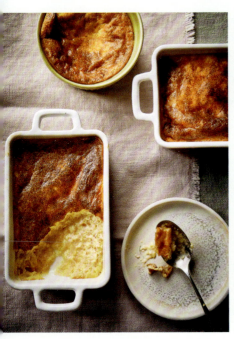
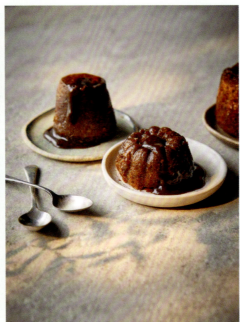
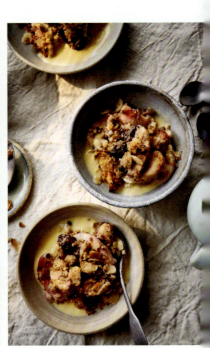

DESSERTS

Lemon Magic Pudding

So-called, as the lemon batter forms its own runny sauce at the bottom of the dish and a light almond sponge on top: genius. So often puddings such as these are extremely high in carbs from the sugar and flour, but I have reduced the sugar to the minimum by using erythritol, which brilliantly balances the sharpness of the lemon. If you would like to do this in advance, mix the lemon cream, but don't touch the egg whites. Cover and leave in the refrigerator for up to a day. When you are ready to cook, take them out of the refrigerator and whisk the egg whites, then continue following the instructions.

1. With the butter, grease 4 ramekins, each around 9 x 4cm (3½ x 1½ inches), or 4 small ovenproof dishes. (If your dishes are shallower than 4cm/1½ inches, allow 8 minutes cooking time.)

2. Put the egg whites into a mixing bowl and set aside. Add all the remaining ingredients to another bowl and use a large spoon to beat them together until they are well blended.

3. Whisk the egg whites until they form stiff peaks.

4. Use a spatula to gently fold the egg whites into the lemon cream. Divide the mixture between the buttered ramekins/dishes and put them on a crisper in the drawer. Air fry the puddings at 160°C (325°F) for 10 minutes, or until golden brown and just firm to the touch. Serve warm.

butter, for greasing
2 eggs, separated
100ml (3½fl oz) double cream
50ml (2fl oz) full-fat milk
50g (1¾oz) erythritol
    or 35g (1¼oz) coconut sugar
35g (1¼oz) ground almonds
finely grated zest and juice of
    ½ lemon
pinch of salt
½ teaspoon baking powder

Per serving with erythritol: 213kcal			
NET CARBS	FIBRE	PROTEIN	FAT
3g	1g	5g	20g
Per serving with sugar: 245kcal			
NET CARBS	FIBRE	PROTEIN	FAT
11g	1g	5g	20g

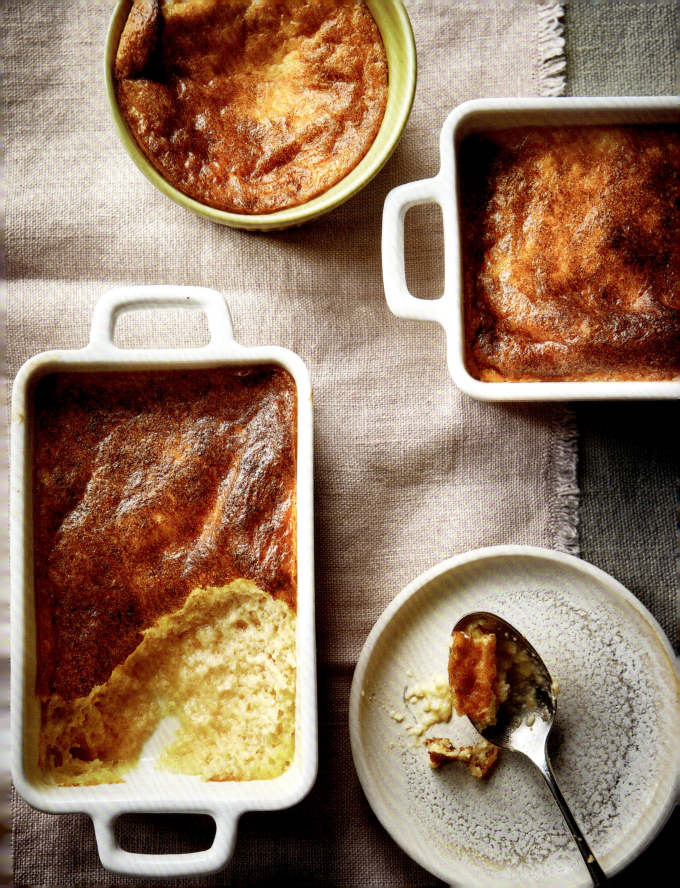

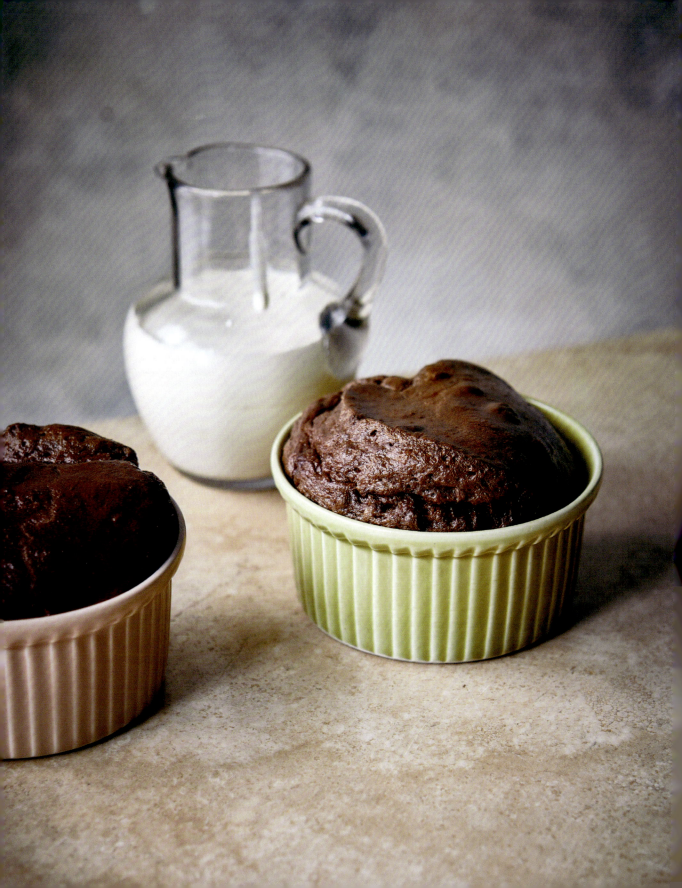

Hot Chocolate Soufflé

This decadent soufflé with a melting middle is just amazing. If you are making this for a dinner party, prepare the custard until it is cooling in a bowl. Leave it in the refrigerator until you are ready, then beat it until smooth, as it will have set firm. Mix it with the egg whites and continue to follow the recipe. Serve these on their own or with Greek yogurt or double cream.

1. Generously butter 4 ramekins, each around 9cm (3½ inches) diameter and 4cm (1½ inches) deep, both inside and around the rim.

2. Put the egg yolks, erythritol, cornflour and vanilla into a small bowl and stir to combine.

3. Pour the milk into a small saucepan and heat until very hot but not boiling. Take a ladleful out and pour this into your egg yolk mixture. Stir through and then add this back into the pan. Whisk until smooth. Continue to heat for a few minutes, stirring constantly over a medium heat until it thickens. Remove from the heat and transfer the custard to a large heatproof bowl straight away. Add the chocolate and stir gently through as it melts.

4. Cool to room temperature. Now is the time to leave the mixture if you don't want to use it yet – cover and put into the refrigerator for up to a day (see intro above).

5. Preheat the air fryer to 160°C (325°F) (on a bake setting, if you have it, for a lower fan speed).

6. Meanwhile, whisk the egg whites to soft peaks in a separate bowl. Take a little of this mixture and use it to loosen the custard in the bowl. Whisk it in to get rid of any lumps. Now gently fold in the rest of the egg whites, keeping as much air in as possible. Spoon the mixture into the prepared ramekins and level the tops. Put the ramekins into the air fryer drawer and cook for 8 minutes until risen.

7. Remove the soufflés from the drawer using an angled slice or silicone tongs and serve straight away with Greek yogurt or cream.

butter, for greasing
4 eggs, separated
20g (¾oz) erythritol or 1 tablespoon coconut or ordinary cane sugar or honey
3 teaspoons (7g/¼oz) cornflour
2 teaspoons vanilla extract
200ml (7fl oz) full-fat milk
80g (2¾oz) dark chocolate (at least 85% cocoa solids), finely chopped or grated

Per serving with erythritol: 215kcal			
NET CARBS	FIBRE	PROTEIN	FAT
11g	0g	9g	16g
Per serving with honey or sugar: 226kcal			
NET CARBS	FIBRE	PROTEIN	FAT
14g	0g	9g	16g

Blackberry and Apple Crumble with Vanilla Custard

Serves 6

You can make this in advance and cook it at the last minute. Prepare the crumble and reheat at 170°C (340°F) covered in tin foil for 5 minutes, then remove the tin foil and continue to cook for 2 minutes, or until browned.

To lower the carb count of the custard by 3g, use almond milk. If you can't eat egg, use ready-made sugar-free custard powder.

1. Put all the filling ingredients along with 100ml (3½fl oz) water into the drawer and air fry at 160°C (325°F) for 25–30 minutes, or until the fruit has softened. Stir a couple of times during cooking.

2. Meanwhile, make the crumble. Add the butter and ground almonds to a mixing bowl and rub them together with your fingertips until they resemble breadcrumbs. Add all the remaining ingredients into the bowl and mix them through, breaking up the flaked almonds a little. Set aside.

3. Put the warm filling into an ovenproof dish or into 6 separate dishes that fit your air fryer drawer. Cover with the crumble topping. Bake at 200°C (400°F) for 3–5 minutes, or until crisp and golden on top. Serve hot with the vanilla custard.

Vanilla Custard

1. Whisk the cornflour into 100ml (3½fl oz) of the milk in a mixing bowl until smooth.

2. Put the date, if using, in 3 tablespoons of the remaining milk in a cup and heat in the microwave on high for 1 minute, or in a pan over a medium heat. It will become soft and can be mashed with a fork. Sieve the mixture into a bowl, pushing it through with the back of a spoon, and whisk. Discard the date skin. Add the egg yolks and whisk until smooth. If using erythritol, add this to the egg yolks.

3. Heat the remaining milk and vanilla in a saucepan until very hot but not boiling. Whisk 2 ladlefuls of hot milk into the egg yolk mixture to bring the temperature of both liquids to a similar heat.

4. Whisk the hot milk in the pan while you pour in the egg mixture. Continue whisking over a medium heat until thickened. Remove from the heat. Serve straight away, or cover the surface with wetted nonstick baking paper to stop it forming a skin. The custard will keep in the refrigerator, covered, for up to 3 days.

For the filling
800g (1lb 12oz) cooking or dessert apples, cored and roughly sliced
200g (7oz) fresh or frozen blackberries
2 tablespoons erythritol or 4 medjool dates, pitted and finely chopped
1 cinnamon stick

For the crumble
25g (1oz) butter, softened
100g (3½oz) ground almonds
50g (1¾oz) flaked almonds
35g (1¼oz) erythritol or 25g (1oz) coconut sugar
1 teaspoon ground cinnamon
½ teaspoon vanilla powder or 1½ teaspoons vanilla extract

Per serving with dates and sugar: 317kcal			
NET CARBS	FIBRE	PROTEIN	FAT
33g	8g	7g	18g
Per serving with erythritol: 273kcal			
NET CARBS	FIBRE	PROTEIN	FAT
21g	7g	7g	18g

15g (½oz) cornflour
500ml (18fl oz) cows' or almond milk
1 fat medjool date (approx. 25g/1oz), pitted and roughly chopped, or 2 tablespoons erythritol
4 egg yolks
2 teaspoons vanilla extract

Per serving with a date: 101kcal			
NET CARBS	FIBRE	PROTEIN	FAT
9g	0g	4g	5g
Per serving with erythritol: 90kcal			
NET CARBS	FIBRE	PROTEIN	FAT
6g	0g	4g	5g

The Diabetes Air Fryer Cookbook

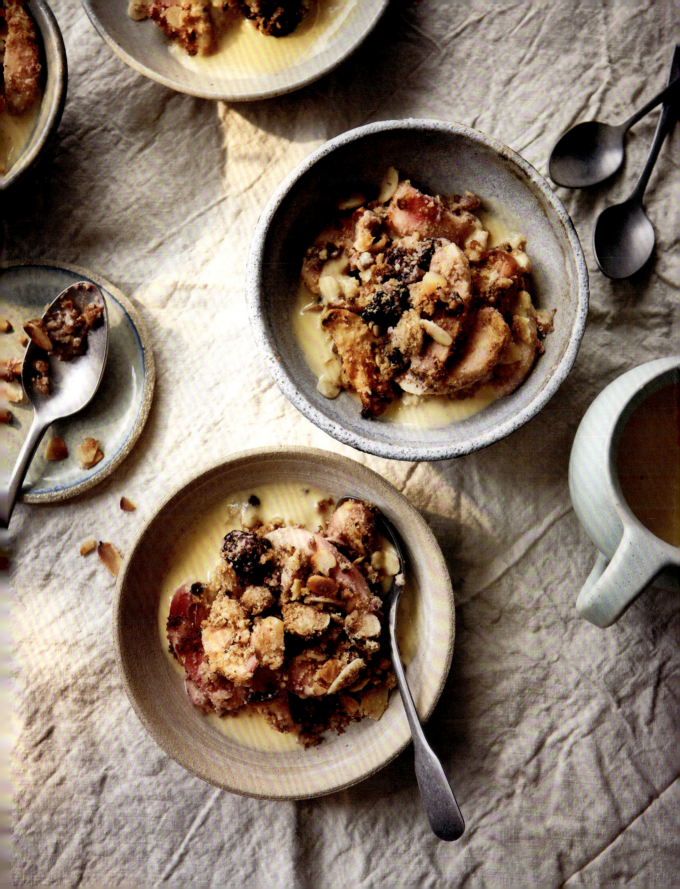

Mini Hazelnut and Chocolate Bites

Makes approx. 16 bites

These are ideal to have after a meal to take away the craving for something sweet. If I have friends visiting, I put these on a wooden board with blackberries, a handful of Granola (see page 34) and thick Greek yogurt dusted with ground cinnamon for dipping. They are small and perfectly formed so are not too calorific or carby. They are great with coffee or tea and to pack up for work and travel. The bites are crunchy when they come out of the air fryer but will soften (due to the reduced sugar levels); to crisp them up, pop them back in the air fryer at 200°C (400°F) for 2 minutes. Alternatively, just think of them as soft cookies!

1. Put a crisper into the drawer and spray or brush it with oil.

2. Toast the hazelnuts on the crisper at 200°C (400°F) for 4 minutes, or until lightly browned. If they still have their thin skins on, rub them in a tea towel to remove the skins. You can also do this in a silicone liner by folding the sides over and rubbing the nuts. Pick out the nuts and discard the skins.

3. Put the nuts in a ziplock bag and bash them with a rolling pin to break them up into the texture of sand and gravel.

4. Tip the nuts into a mixing bowl with all the the remaining ingredients and stir through until combined. Use a teaspoon to drop approx. 8–10g (¼oz) pieces of the mixture on the oiled crisper, keeping them 1cm (½ inch) apart. You may have to do this in batches.

5. Air fry at 140°C (275°F) for 10 minutes, or until browned and firm to the touch. Remove from the air fryer and allow to cool to room temperature on a wire rack before serving.

extra-virgin olive oil
50g (1¾oz) hazelnuts or walnuts, pecans or almonds, or a mixture
1 tablespoon erythritol or 2 teaspoons honey
1 tablespoon coconut flour
15g (½oz) butter, softened
1 egg white
1 teaspoon vanilla extract
15g (½oz) dark chocolate (at least 85% cocoa solids), finely chopped

Per bite with erythritol: 36kcal			
NET CARBS	FIBRE	PROTEIN	FAT
1g	0.5g	1g	3g
Per bite with honey: 39kcal			
NET CARBS	FIBRE	PROTEIN	FAT
1.5g	0.5g	1g	3g

The Diabetes Air Fryer Cookbook

Raspberry Heart Cookies

Eat these cookies as they are or crumble them over yogurt, cream or fruit. They become soft after a day but can easily be re-baked in the air fryer for a couple of minutes to firm up.

1. Spray or brush a crisper in the drawer with oil.

2. Cut 6 of the larger raspberries in half for the filling of the cookies and set aside. Put all the remaining ingredients into a bowl and use a metal spoon to stir them together until combined, breaking up the raspberries as you go.

3. Use a teaspoon to pick up a walnut-sized ball of the mixture, and roll it gently between your hands. Flatten the ball of dough and put half a raspberry inside the ball. Bring the edges up and around it and seal it into a ball. Flatten it gently. It should be approx. 5cm (2 inches) wide and 1.5cm (⅝ inch) thick. Put it on the oiled crisper in the drawer and repeat with the rest of the dough and raspberry halves, leaving a finger-width gap between them. You may need to do this in batches.

4. Bake at 160°C (325°F) for 8 minutes, or until golden brown and firm to the touch. Continue rolling and cooking in batches until all the cookies are done. Transfer the cookies by carefully lifting them with a silicone spatula on to a wire rack. Leave to cool to room temperature.

5. Serve straight away, or store in an airtight container for up to 2 days at room temperature or for up to 5 days in the refrigerator. If they become soft, re-bake them at 160°C (325°F) for up to 3 minutes to firm up.

Tips and tricks

Instead of the raspberry filling, mix 10g (¼oz) dark chocolate chips (at least 85% cocoa solids) into the mixture before shaping and baking.

extra-virgin olive oil
150g (5½oz) fresh raspberries
2 eggs
10g (¼oz) erythritol or 2 teaspoons honey
10g (¼oz) coconut oil or softened butter
65g (2¼oz) coconut flour

Per cookie with erythritol: 44kcal			
NET CARBS	FIBRE	PROTEIN	FAT
2g	2g	2g	2g
Per cookie with honey: 48kcal			
NET CARBS	FIBRE	PROTEIN	FAT
3g	2g	2g	2g

Roast Strawberries and Lime Cheesecake Cream with Crumble

This indulgent dessert can be made quickly when strawberries are in season. It's also a great way to use up strawberries just past their best. Use a mixture or just one type of berry. Look out for pure cream cheese, not one with additives. Luckily this is often the cheapest own-brand variety. Orange or lemon zest are gorgeous with this, if you don't have lime for the cream.

1. Put the berries into a silicone liner or ovenproof container and add the orange zest. Add 3 tablespoons of water and 1 teaspoon of the vanilla and then stir through. Air fry at 200°C (400°F) for 8–10 minutes, or until the berries are soft, stirring halfway through.

2. Whisk all the remaining ingredients together in a bowl using an electric whisk or balloon whisk until you have a smooth cream. Chill in the refrigerator until needed.

3. Make the crumble. Add the butter and ground almonds to a mixing bowl and rub them together with your fingertips until they resemble breadcrumbs. Add all the remaining ingredients into the bowl and mix them through, breaking up the flaked almonds a little. Air fry the crumble in a silicone liner at 180°C (350°F) for 5–7 minutes until golden brown, tossing the mixture halfway through. Do keep an eye on it, as it can burn quickly. Transfer the crumble to a large plate to cool.

4. To serve, shallow bowls are ideal; spoon the cheesecake cream on to one side of each bowl and the strawberries on to the other. Scatter the crumble over the cream and serve straight away.

500g (1lb 2oz) fresh berries (such as strawberries, raspberries, blackberries, blueberries or currants), large ones halved
finely grated zest of ½ orange
2 teaspoons vanilla extract
150g (5½oz) Greek yogurt
150g (5½oz) cream cheese
finely grated zest of 1 lime
1 heaped tablespoon (15g/½oz) erythritol or 1 tablespoon honey

For the crumble
15g (½oz) butter, softened
50g (1¾oz) ground almonds
25g (1oz) flaked almonds
20g (¾oz) erythritol or 15g (½oz) coconut sugar
¼ teaspoon vanilla powder or ¾ teaspoon vanilla extract

Per serving of strawberries and cheese-cake cream with erythritol: 181kcal			
NET CARBS	FIBRE	PROTEIN	FAT
10g	3g	5g	14g
Per serving of strawberries and cheesecake cream with honey: 192kcal			
NET CARBS	FIBRE	PROTEIN	FAT
13g	3g	5g	14g

Per serving of crumble with erythritol: 189kcal			
NET CARBS	FIBRE	PROTEIN	FAT
2g	2g	6g	17g
Per serving of crumble with sugar: 204kcal			
NET CARBS	FIBRE	PROTEIN	FAT
6g	2g	6g	17g

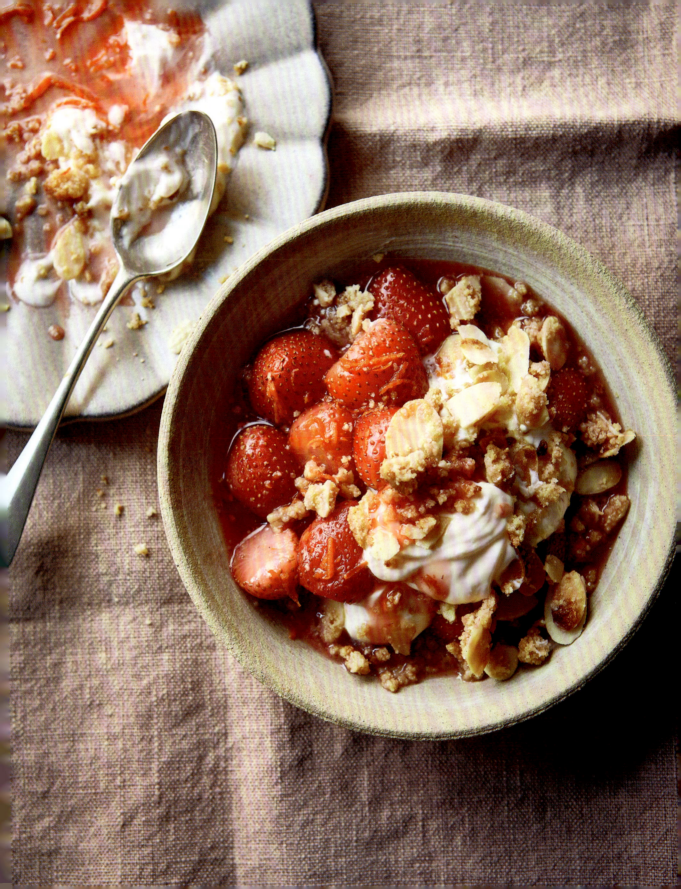

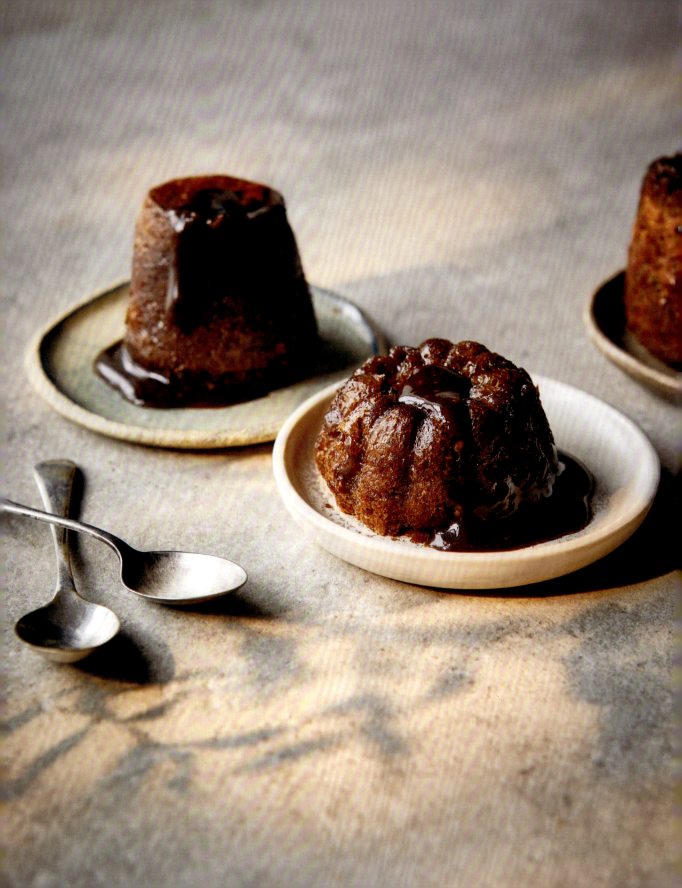

Sticky Toffee Pudding

Although we've reduced the carbs by almost half in this popular British pudding, to change the recipe any further would take it too far from the original. Therefore, this is a treat and a delicious one that won't leave you feeling like you can't move off the sofa for the rest of the day.

Black treacle is a mixture of molasses and sugar syrup. Its distinct flavour gives a smoky bittersweet flavour to this pudding. You can replace it with erythritol but the flavour will be very different. Dates are essential in the sponge for flavour and texture.

1. To make the sauce, put 50ml (2fl oz) water into a small pan and add the chopped date. Add the treacle, cream and butter, place over a medium heat and bring the mixture to the boil, then cook, stirring, until the butter melts. Remove from the heat and mash the date using a potato masher or a stick blender. Replace the pan over the heat and keep cooking for a few minutes until it thickens. Set aside while you make the puddings. This step can be done in advance; the sauce will keep in the refrigerator for up to 2 days (if the sauce is cold, warm it in a small pan to use).

2. Generously grease 4 metal 6 x 6cm (2½ x 2½ inch) deep dariole moulds or 9 x 4cm (3½ x 1½ inch) deep ramekins with butter. Or use 6 smaller, 7 x 4cm (2¾ x 1½ inch) deep fluted moulds.

3. To make the puddings, soften the dates in 75ml (2½fl oz) very hot water in a small bowl.

4. Put all the ingredients for the pudding, including the dates and their soaking water, into a small blender, or use a stick blender in a bowl, and purée until smooth. If you don't have a blender, mash the dates into the water with a fork and then add the remaining ingredients and beat together with a wooden spoon.

5. Divide the pudding mixture between the prepared moulds. Place the moulds into the air fryer drawer and bake the puddings at 170°C (340°F) for 10 minutes until risen and firm to the touch.

6. Remove the puddings from the drawer with tongs or an angled slice and leave them to sit for 5 minutes.

7. Meanwhile, warm the sauce gently in a small pan over a medium heat. Run a knife around the rim of each pudding and use a cloth or oven gloves to turn out the puddings on serving plates. Top each one with the sauce, and serve on their own or with double cream.

For the sauce
1 fat medjool date (approx. 25g/1oz), pitted and roughly chopped
1 teaspoon black treacle
75ml (2½fl oz) double cream
25g (1oz) butter

For the pudding
butter, for greasing
2 fat medjool dates (approx. 50g/1¾oz), pitted and roughly chopped
2 eggs
60g (2¼oz) ground almonds
1 teaspoon bicarbonate of soda
2 teaspoons (10g/¼oz) black treacle
2 teaspoons vanilla extract
small pinch of salt

Per serving of sauce for 4: 157kcal			
NET CARBS	FIBRE	PROTEIN	FAT
5g	0g	1g	15g
Per serving of pudding for 4: 167kcal			
NET CARBS	FIBRE	PROTEIN	FAT
12g	2g	6g	11g

Per serving of sauce for 6: 104kcal			
NET CARBS	FIBRE	PROTEIN	FAT
4g	0g	0g	10g
Per serving of pudding for 6: 111kcal			
NET CARBS	FIBRE	PROTEIN	FAT
7g	1g	4g	7g

Pears in Red Wine

This traditional Italian winter dish is usually loaded with sugar, but in this version I have used erythritol and the natural sweetness of raspberries instead. The speed of the air fryer reduces the cooking time to just 30 minutes from an hour. Double or triple the quantity for a special dinner; everything can be made in advance and reheated at 160°C (325°F) for around 15 minutes in an ovenproof dish or a silicone liner in the air fryer.

    Following our idea of having smaller portions, this serves half a pear per person, and actually it is enough.

1. Put the pear and the other ingredients into an ovenproof dish in which they fit snugly. Put the dish in the drawer and bake them in the air fryer at 160°C (325°F) for 30 minutes.

2. Remove and discard the cloves and transfer the pear halves to 2 serving dishes.

3. Put the sauce into a container and blitz with a stick blender or push it through a sieve to thicken the sauce.

4. Pour over the pears while still warm and serve with mascarpone or double cream.

1 pear, peeled and halved lengthways
150ml (5fl oz) red wine
2 cloves
1 heaped tablespoon (15g/½oz) erythritol or 1 tablespoon honey
35g (1¼oz) raspberries
mascarpone or double cream, to serve

Tips and tricks
Finely grate orange zest or chocolate over the top for a decadent finish.

Per serving with erythritol: 123kcal			
NET CARBS	FIBRE	PROTEIN	FAT
14g	4g	1g	0g
Per serving with honey: 147kcal			
NET CARBS	FIBRE	PROTEIN	FAT
20g	4g	1g	0g

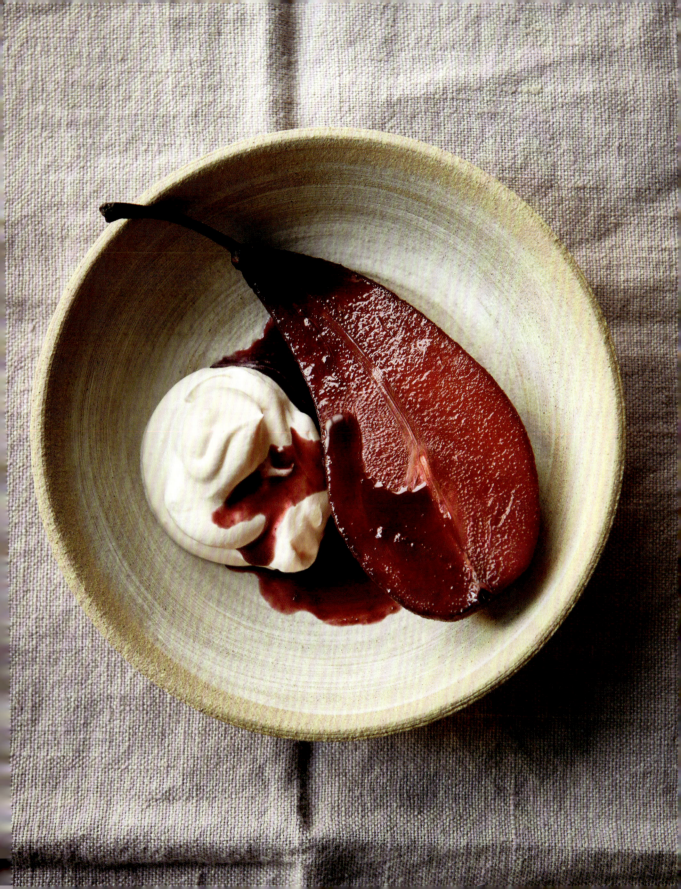

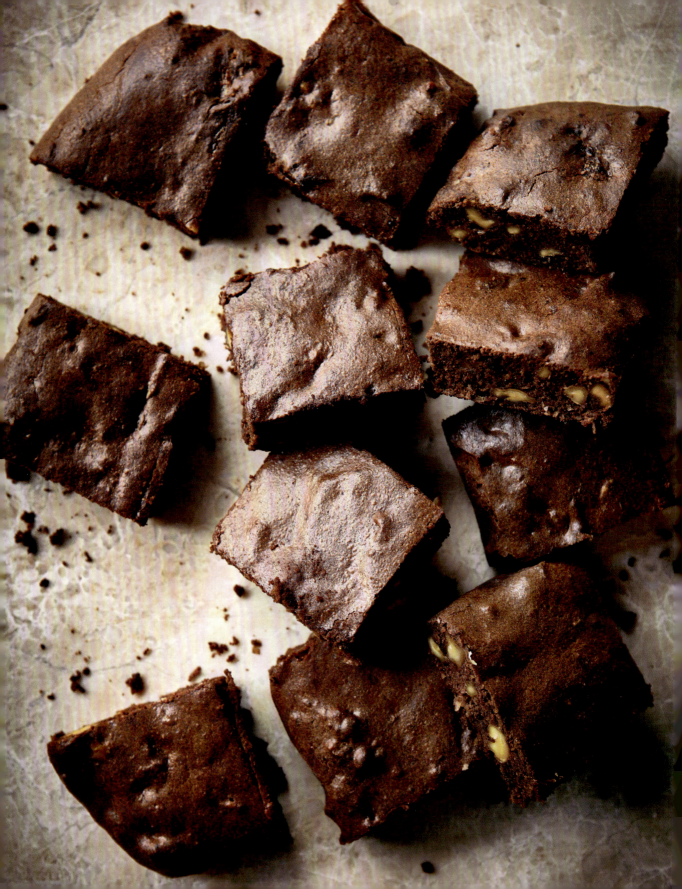

Stefano's Squidgy Chocolate, Date and Walnut Brownies

Stefano is the Head Chef of our cookery school and has created this recipe to have minimal sweetness and maximum flavour. They are also full of fibre from the nuts, chocolate and dates. Toasting nuts brings out the natural oils and gives them oodles of flavour. Smell them as they go into the air fryer and come out and you will see what I mean. If you are keeping your carbs very low, use erythritol instead of the dates.

Leave these plain, top with whipped cream flavoured with vanilla or serve with Greek yogurt, crème fraîche or soured cream, and berries.

1. Toast the walnuts on a crisper in the drawer at 160°C (325°F) for 3 minutes. Tip them out to cool before roughly chopping them.

2. If using the dates, soak them in 75ml (2½fl oz) of just-boiled water for a few minutes, then mash them to a pulp with a fork. If using erythritol, dissolve it in 50ml (2fl oz) of just-boiled water in a small saucepan over a medium-high heat. Set aside.

3. Put a baking paper liner into a silicone liner.

4. Melt the chocolate and butter together in a bain-marie (a glass or metal bowl over, but not touching, hot water in a saucepan over a medium heat) or in a small bowl in the microwave. Set aside to cool.

5. Separate the eggs into 2 mixing bowls. Add the date or erythritol mixture to the egg yolks and stir through with a hand whisk or large spoon. Then add the chocolate mixture to the yolk mixture with the walnuts and ground almonds and stir again to combine.

6. Whisk the egg whites until just firm enough to stand in peaks. Use a large metal spoon to fold the egg whites into the chocolate mixture. Pour into the prepared liner and smooth the surface.

7. Bake in the air fryer at 140°C (275°F) for 20–25 minutes. It is ready when the crust feels firm but there should be a slight wobble to it; it will continue setting as it cools. Remove from the air fryer and leave to cool to room temperature before removing from the paper liner.

8. Cut into 12 squares and serve at room temperature. Or put into an airtight container in the refrigerator once cool, where they will keep for a couple of days.

75g (2½oz) walnuts
3 fat medjool dates (approx. 75g/2½oz), pitted and roughly chopped, or 75g (2½oz) erythritol
100g (3½oz) dark chocolate (at least 85% cocoa solids)
60g (2¼oz) butter, plus extra for greasing
3 eggs
50g (1¾oz) ground almonds

Per brownie with dates: 181kcal			
NET CARBS	FIBRE	PROTEIN	FAT
5g	2g	4g	16g
Per brownie with erythritol: 171kcal			
NET CARBS	FIBRE	PROTEIN	FAT
3g	2g	4g	16g

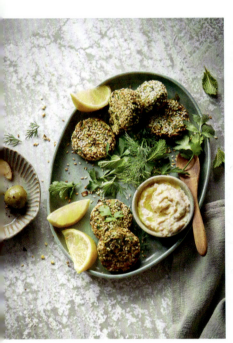

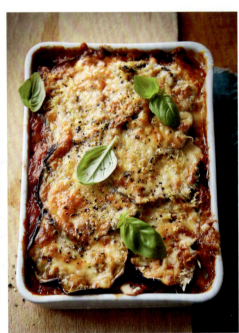

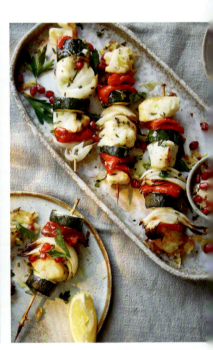

HELPER RECIPES

Hummus

Everyone loves this creamy dip yet so many people buy it when it is easy to make at home. By making your own you can decide the best oil to use and season it as you like. To make it vegan, replace the yogurt with water.

1. Put all the ingredients, apart from 6 whole chickpeas, into a food processor and whizz until creamy, adding a little water as necessary. Adjust to taste with lemon juice, tahini or seasoning. Spoon into a serving dish.

2. Pour a little olive oil on top of the hummus and use the back of a spoon to flatten it and spread over the olive oil. This does two things: it makes it look glossy and attractive and protects the surface from becoming dry. Scatter the reserved chickpeas and the sumac, if using, on top.

400g (14oz) can chickpeas, drained (240g/8½oz drained weight)
75ml (2½fl oz) extra-virgin olive oil, plus 2 teaspoons for drizzling
1 garlic clove
2 tablespoons lemon juice, or more to taste
2 tablespoons tahini, or more to taste
½ teaspoon salt
¼ teaspoon freshly ground black pepper
½ teaspoon sumac, to serve (optional)

Per serving: 278kcal			
NET CARBS	FIBRE	PROTEIN	FAT
5g	5g	6g	25g

Guacamole

Guacamole should be made out of perfectly ripe avocados, preferably the dark green, bumpy-skinned Hass variety, as they have a good flavour and creamy texture. It is great with chicken, carrot sticks, or heaped on halved boiled eggs or low-carb bread.

Leave out the chilli as you wish, but if you are adding it, taste it first, and remember the heat is in the pith and not the seeds. Try a tiny piece from the centre of the chilli – the ends are usually milder.

1. Mash the avocados with a fork in a bowl. Add all the remaining ingredients, then taste and adjust the salt and chilli for the balance of seasoning and heat. Guacamole will keep in the refrigerator, covered, for a couple of days.

flesh of 2 ripe Hass avocados
juice of 1½ limes
½–¾ teaspoon salt
small handful of fresh coriander, finely chopped
⅛–¼ jalapeño chilli or ¼–½ red chilli, finely chopped, or Tabasco sauce, to taste
1 small garlic clove, finely chopped
1 tomato, diced

Per serving: 81kcal			
NET CARBS	FIBRE	PROTEIN	FAT
2g	3g	1g	7g

Cucumber Raita

This creamy, refreshing dip is perfect for cooling spicy dishes. Swap the coriander for parsley for coriander-haters!

1. Mix all the ingredients together in a bowl with a spoon. Taste and adjust the seasoning.

2. Transfer to a serving bowl, cover and keep chilled until you are ready to serve. It will keep for up to a day in the refrigerator.

150g (5½oz) Greek yogurt
½ long cucumber, diced
10g (¼oz) mint leaves, finely chopped
7g (¼oz) fresh coriander or parsley leaves, finely chopped
1 teaspoon ground cumin
2 tablespoons lemon juice
salt
a few fresh coriander leaves, to serve

Per serving: 54kcal			
NET CARBS	FIBRE	PROTEIN	FAT
2g	0.5g	2g	4g

One-minute Mayonnaise

Take your pick as to which oil to use from the list below, but don't be tempted to use extra-virgin olive oil in this mayo; it is too strong and bitter. Like most homemade mayonnaises, this is made with raw egg. This is the basic recipe, but you can flavour it with a little grated fresh garlic, finely grated lemon zest, chopped chives or chipotle or curry powder.

1. Put all the ingredients into the narrow, tall mixing bowl of a stick blender. If you don't have one, use a tall, narrow jam jar instead. There should be only up to 1cm (½ inch) of room around the base of the blender stick.

2. Push the stick blender to the bottom, beneath the egg and whizz for 15 seconds, or until you see a thick mayonnaise forming. At that point, while mixing, slowly lift the blender upward to mix all the oil in.

3. Now taste the mayonnaise; at this point you can stir in more mustard, lemon juice, seasoning or other flavourings. It will keep, covered, for up to 3 days in the refrigerator.

1 medium egg
1 heaped teaspoon Dijon mustard, or more to taste
1 teaspoon lemon juice, or more to taste
½ teaspoon salt, or more to taste
good few twists of freshly ground black pepper, or more to taste
150ml (5fl oz) cold pressed rapeseed oil, avocado, macadamia or light olive oil

Per serving: 54kcal			
NET CARBS	FIBRE	PROTEIN	FAT
0.5g	0g	1g	39g

Tips and tricks

Garlic mayonnaise: Simply add ½–1 teaspoon of grated garlic to the mayonnaise, to taste.

Classic Tomato Sauce

This is an easy tomato sauce to make from canned peeled tomatoes. Always choose an Italian variety; either San Marzano plum tomatoes or cherry tomatoes are perfect. This will keep in the refrigerator for up to 5 days and can be frozen for up to 3 months. This is perfect for Gloria's Meatballs (see page 114) or with a pasta alternative such as Buttered Cabbage Ribbons (see page 147).

1. Heat the olive oil in a pan over a medium heat and fry the onion and garlic for 5–7 minutes until softened and translucent. Season with salt and pepper.

2. Add the tomatoes and rinse the cans out with a little water, then add this to the pan. Bash the tomatoes with a potato masher or wooden spoon to break them up. Reduce the heat and simmer, uncovered, for about 40 minutes to concentrate the flavours. The sauce should be thick and not watery. Taste and adjust the seasoning as necessary.

4 tablespoons extra-virgin olive oil
1 red or white onion (approx. 200g/7oz), finely chopped
2 garlic cloves
3 x 400g (14oz) cans Italian plum tomatoes
salt and pepper

Tips and tricks

Protein-packed tomato pasta:
Usually, the classic dish of pasta and tomato sauce is loaded with carbs and lacking in protein. However, see my easy tip on page 124 using silken tofu to add a creamy texture while bumping up the protein. I usually suggest serving the sauce over green vegetables rather than pasta, but for an extra protein hit you can mix veggies with a small portion (around 25g/1oz dried weight) of protein-rich pasta such as spinach farfalle or red lentil pasta, but watch how the carbs increase.

Per serving: 127kcal			
NET CARBS	FIBRE	PROTEIN	FAT
9g	4g	2g	10g

Per serving of tomato sauce with tofu: 189kcal			
NET CARBS	FIBRE	PROTEIN	FAT
11g	4g	9g	12g

Per serving serving of tomato sauce with added tofu and lentil pasta: 279kcal			
NET CARBS	FIBRE	PROTEIN	FAT
25g	6g	16g	13g

Onion Gravy

By using the air fryer you can have sweet, fried onions in just 15 minutes. I am all in favour of collecting meat fat and juices leftover from a roast to make dripping just as my mother and grandmother did before me. It is useful cooking fat, and free, and is full of flavour. Many onion gravies are sweetened with sugar or jam, but here I use erythritol.

1. Put the onion, both the fats, the herbs and some seasoning in the drawer or in an ovenproof dish. Air fry at 180°C (350°F) for 15 minutes, or until soft and lightly browned, stirring twice to make sure all the onion is covered in fat.

2. Add the wine to the drawer and stir it through the onion with a spatula. Pour the mixture into a saucepan over a medium-high heat. Bring to a bubbling boil and let it reduce for around 4 minutes, or until the strong smell of wine has gone.

3. Add the balsamic vinegar and the stock and stir through. Continue to cook again, letting it bubble vigorously for 5 minutes.

4. In a small bowl, mix the cornflour with a teaspoon of water. Stir into the gravy. Season to taste with the erythritol and more seasoning as necessary. Pour into a warm jug to serve.

1 white onion, finely chopped
1 tablespoon dripping or extra-virgin olive oil
25g (1oz) butter or more dripping
2 thyme sprigs or 1 teaspoon dried thyme leaves
200ml (7fl oz) red wine
2 teaspoons balsamic vinegar
400ml (14fl oz) hot chicken stock or water
2 teaspoons cornflour
1 tablespoon erythritol or 2 teaspoons mild honey, or to taste
salt and pepper

Per serving with erythritol: 105kcal			
NET CARBS	FIBRE	PROTEIN	FAT
6g	1g	1g	6g
Per serving with honey: 112kcal			
NET CARBS	FIBRE	PROTEIN	FAT
8g	1g	1g	6g

Vegetable Mash

Root vegetables, brassicas and squashes that aren't high in carbs are perfect for making a delicious rainbow of mash with a fraction of the carbs compared to potato mash. Swede mash, for example, contains 3g of carbs per serving, whereas potato mash has 16g. Celeriac goes well with meat as well as fish; while cauliflower, Brussels sprouts and swede work better with meat, sausages and eggs. Pumpkin is also good, but butternut squash and parsnip are too high in carbs for low-carbers. The vegetables can be mashed with a potato masher, but a food processor or stick blender gives the creamy texture that we all love. Any leftovers will keep well in the refrigerator for up to 3 days, and make a good base for eggs the next day.

By using the leaves and stalks of the brassicas you get a lot more mash. Cut the stalks into smaller pieces than the rest of the vegetables and cook first. Add the leaves last to ensure even cooking.

Some vegetables are more absorbent than others, so you will need to alter the milk quantity accordingly.

1. Steam or boil the vegetables in a pan of boiling water until just tender, then drain.

2. Tip into a food processor, along with all the remaining ingredients and blend until you have a soft, smooth mash. Alternatively, blend using a stick blender. Taste and adjust the seasoning as necessary. Spoon into a warm bowl and dot with extra butter to serve.

Tips and tricks

Mix leftover cooked veg from your refrigerator into the mash. One of our favourite combos is leek and cauliflower.

400g (14oz) prepared low-carb vegetable/s such as Brussels sprouts, cauliflower, swede, pumpkin, celeriac, broccoli
25g (1oz) salted butter or extra-virgin olive oil, plus extra to serve
25–75ml (1–2½fl oz) cows' milk, double cream or crème fraîche
½ teaspoon ground nutmeg (optional)
salt and pepper

Per serving of Brussels sprout mash: 91kcal			
NET CARBS	FIBRE	PROTEIN	FAT
5g	4g	4g	5g

Per serving of cauliflower mash: 74kcal			
NET CARBS	FIBRE	PROTEIN	FAT
3g	2g	2g	5g

Per serving of swede mash: 60kcal			
NET CARBS	FIBRE	PROTEIN	FAT
3g	0.5g	1g	5g

Per serving of pumpkin mash: 68kcal			
NET CARBS	FIBRE	PROTEIN	FAT
4g	1g	1g	5g

Per serving of celeriac mash: 90kcal			
NET CARBS	FIBRE	PROTEIN	FAT
8g	2g	2g	5g

Per serving of broccoli mash: 82kcal			
NET CARBS	FIBRE	PROTEIN	FAT
4g	3g	3g	5g

Cauliflower Rice

To avoid the spikes of glucose in your bloodstream from eating rice or couscous, switch to cauliflower rice. It takes just 10 minutes to prepare and has endless flavour possibilities. I stir-fry it with onion, which gives a wonderful taste. Eat it just like this or add other flavours, such as chopped fresh coriander or cumin seeds. Once cooked, it keeps well in the refrigerator for up to 3 days (or in the freezer for up to 3 months). You can use broccoli or Brussels sprouts in the same way.

1. Put one-third of the cauliflower into a food processor and pulse until finely chopped (it will resemble large grains of rice), making sure you don't end up with a purée. Tip the cauliflower into a bowl and repeat with the remaining two-thirds. If you don't have a food processor, coarsely grate the cauliflower florets and stalk and finely chop the leaves.

2. Heat the oil in a wok or large frying pan. Fry the onion over a medium heat for 5–7 minutes, or until soft. Add the cauliflower rice, season and stir through. Add 75ml (2½fl oz) water, cover and cook over a low heat for about 7 minutes or until just soft, stirring occasionally, then serve.

200g (7oz) cauliflower or broccoli, head cut into large florets, stalk and leaves roughly chopped, or Brussels sprouts, trimmed
1 tablespoon extra-virgin olive oil (or ghee, coconut oil, chicken fat or beef dripping)
1 small onion (or leek), or 5 spring onions, finely chopped
salt and pepper

Per serving: 52kcal			
NET CARBS	FIBRE	PROTEIN	FAT
4g	2g	2g	3g

My Perfect Green Salad with Fresh Herbs and Vinaigrette

Serves 4

Sometimes a burst of one colour can be just as dramatic as a rainbow. I love to use my imagination, seeing what I can throw into a salad while keeping it green. Below is a guide, not a prescription. If you have only one kind of salad leaf and dislike pepper, no problem, it will be your perfect salad.

1. Prepare the salad in a large serving bowl and add the vinaigrette (to taste) at the last minute.

You will need approx. 600g (1lb 5oz) of your favourite green salad ingredients; this is my selection:

1 large or 2 medium spring onions, trimmed, finely chopped
1 fennel bulb, trimmed and thinly sliced
½ long cucumber, peeled and cubed
1 green pepper, cored, deseeded and cut into thin strips
1 ripe avocado, peeled, stone removed, cubed
sweet lettuce, such as little gem, roughly torn
bitter leaves, such as chicory or romaine, roughly torn
spicy leaves, such as watercress, rocket or cress
100g (3½oz) mangetout or sugar snap peas, halved
a large handful of basil or mint leaves, or both
1 quantity of Vinaigrette (see below)

Per serving: 60kcal			
NET CARBS	FIBRE	PROTEIN	FAT
4g	4g	2g	3g

Vinaigrette

Serves 4

My earliest memory of cooking is from when I was around 6 years old. My job was to shake vinaigrette dressing in a jar for my mum as she prepared salad for us all. She would get me to taste it and decide if it needed more of any of the ingredients. In that simple task she gave me confidence in my ability to taste. Thanks Mum.

1. Put all the ingredients in a jar and shake until emulsified. Taste it and ask yourself or a small child if you/they like it! Adjust with extra salt, mustard or lemon juice as necessary. Keep any leftover dressing the sealed jar in the refrigerator for up to a week.

1 tablespoon red wine vinegar
4 tablespoons extra-virgin olive oil
¼ teaspoon salt, or more if needed
good pinch of freshly ground black pepper
1 teaspoon Dijon mustard, or more if needed
1 teaspoon lemon juice, or more if needed
1 small garlic clove, grated (optional)
1 heaped teaspoon erythritol or ½ teaspoon honey (optional)

Per serving with honey: 121kcal			
NET CARBS	FIBRE	PROTEIN	FAT
1g	0g	0g	14g
Per serving with erythritol: 105kcal			
NET CARBS	FIBRE	PROTEIN	FAT
0g	0g	0g	14g

Super Simple Tuscan Salad

Serves 2

Giancarlo loves quartered ripe, flavourful tomatoes simply dressed with basil, oil and salt. He will eat them with any meal, from scrambled eggs in the morning to a steak at night. This salad is quick to prepare. You can make it a couple of hours in advance, but don't add the dressing until the last minute, as the salt makes the tomatoes soft.

1. Soak the diced onion in a bowl of cold water for 15 minutes.

2. Put the oil and vinegar together in a serving bowl and season lightly with a pinch of salt and pepper. Stir them together.

3. Cut away and discard the cores of the tomatoes and then cut them into wedges. If using cherry tomatoes, simply halve them along the equator rather than pole to pole. Add the tomatoes to the dressing. Drain the onion well in a sieve and then add this and the cucumber and basil to the dressing.

4. Toss the salad with your hands or tongs and serve straight away.

1 spring onion or ½ small red onion, finely diced
1 tablespoon extra-virgin olive oil
1 teaspoon red wine vinegar
200g (7oz) ripe tomatoes
½ long cucumber, peeled and roughly diced
10 basil leaves, roughly torn
salt and pepper

Per serving: 88kcal			
NET CARBS	FIBRE	PROTEIN	FAT
4g	2g	1g	7g

Sweetheart Cabbage and Carrot Slaw

Serves 4

This creamy coleslaw is perfectly matched with the Spicy Buffalo Wings on page 96. You can use any member of the cabbage family to make up the volume. I like to change it up with a chopped green chilli for a kick, fennel instead of cabbage or throw in 25g (1oz) chopped fresh coriander – using up whatever I have in the refrigerator.

1. Combine the mayonnaise, vinegar, lemon juice, mustard, yogurt and seasoning together in a large mixing bowl. Add all the remaining ingredients and stir through to combine.

2. Serve straight away or cover and chill for up to a day before serving.

40g (1½oz) mayonnaise (see page 195 for homemade)
1 tablespoon cider or wine vinegar
2 teaspoons lemon juice or more cider vinegar
1 heaped teaspoon Dijon mustard
25g (1oz) Greek yogurt
250g (9oz) green sweetheart, white or red cabbage, finely shredded
1 carrot (75g/2½oz), coarsely grated
1 celery stick, finely chopped
3 spring onions, finely chopped
salt and pepper

Per serving: 105kcal			
NET CARBS	FIBRE	PROTEIN	FAT
5g	2g	2g	8g

Turkish Chopped Salad

Serves 4

Our Turkish friend Çağlar whips up this traditional salad when we run our wellness retreats in Türkiye each year. He uses his own homemade pomegranate molasses and homegrown lemons. It seems to go with almost everything! Try it with grilled salmon, chicken, steak, the kebabs recipe (see page 120), feta cheese or soft-boiled eggs. Sometimes Çağlar serves this with chopped walnuts for extra protein and crunch factor.

1. Make the dressing by mixing all the ingredients together in a serving bowl and season to taste.

2. Now get chopping, but don't spend ages doing this, as a rough cut is fine. Using a serrated knife, cut the tomatoes into dice, then add to the dressing. Peel the cucumber and dice it. Add to the dressing. Chop the spring onions into fine dice. Add to the dressing.

3. I find the easiest way to cut the lettuce is to lay down the leaves and put the herbs on top (including the stalks but not tough mint stems). Roll them up and hold down with one hand as you chop with the other, cutting them into fine shreds. Add to the dressing, along with the chilli, if using

4. Toss the salad together and taste once more for seasoning before serving.

2 tomatoes or a handful of cherry tomatoes
½ long cucumber
4 spring onions or 1 small onion
small handful (approx. 100g/3½oz) of crunchy salad leaves, such as romaine, iceberg or little gem or watercress
20g (¾oz) mixture of dill, mint leaves, fresh coriander and/or flat leaf parsley
spicy green chilli, finely chopped, or chilli flakes, to taste (optional)

For the dressing
2 tablespoons lemon juice, or to taste
1 tablespoon pomegranate molasses
2 tablespoons extra-virgin olive oil
1 small garlic clove, grated
1 teaspoon sumac (optional)
salt and pepper

Per serving: 94kcal			
NET CARBS	FIBRE	PROTEIN	FAT
6g	2g	1g	7g

Giorgio's Chilli Sauce

Serves 6 (makes approx. 225g/8oz)

This sauce keeps well in a jar in the refrigerator for up to a week.

1. Put all the ingredients into a small food processor and whizz together until smooth. Alternatively, finely chop the chilli(es), grate the tomato and stir together with the rest of the ingredients. Taste and adjust the heat (with more chilli or more kefir/yogurt) and salt as necessary.

2. Use straight away or keep in an airtight container, refrigerated, for up to a week.

1–2 hot red chillies, or more to taste, destemmed
1 small tomato
pinch of dried chilli flakes (optional)
2 tablespoons extra-virgin olive oil
1 tablespoon tahini
½ teaspoon salt, or more to taste
3–5 tablespoons kefir or Greek yogurt, or more to taste
1 teaspoon black onion (nigella) seeds
1 tablespoon pomegranate molasses or 2 teaspoons lemon juice plus 1 teaspoon honey

Per serving: 80kcal			
NET CARBS	FIBRE	PROTEIN	FAT
4g	1g	1g	7g

Tuscan Ragù

Serves 8 (makes approx. 1.6kg/3lb 8oz)

This traditional ragù (meat and tomato sauce for pasta) is a rich, sticky, full-flavoured sauce. It is so useful to have in the refrigerator or freezer, as not only is it gorgeous with the Buttered Cabbage Ribbons on page 147, but also it forms the base of the Cottage Pie, Quick Cheesy Mince, Moussaka, and Lasagne with Ragù and Courgette Layers (see pages 110–111). It will keep in a sealed container in the freezer for up to 3 months.

It is *all about the base*, the 'soffrito', which is a colourful fried, mixture of carrot, onion and celery. You can make this ragù with defrosted frozen minced beef, lamb or pork, or make it vegetarian by simply substituting the minced meat for cooked lentils or roasted vegetables (although the protein would be lower and the carbs higher).

1. Heat the oil in a saucepan over a medium heat and fry the vegetables, garlic and rosemary with seasoning (go easy on the salt if you are using Worcestershire sauce later for the Cottage Pie, see page 111) for around 15 minutes, or until they start to soften, stirring frequently.

2. Add the minced beef to the pan and cook, stirring once, for 10–15 minutes until the beef has browned and most of the water has evaporated. Pour in the red wine and cook for a further 5 minutes to cook off the alcohol. Add the tomatoes and purée, stir through and cook, uncovered, for 1 hour until the mixture has reduced and thickened.

3. Taste and adjust the seasoning to your liking.

4 tablespoons extra-virgin olive oil
1 onion, finely chopped
1 carrot, finely chopped
2 celery sticks, finely chopped
1 fat garlic clove, lightly crushed with the flat of a knife
1 rosemary sprig or ½ teaspoon dried rosemary
1kg (2lb 4oz) minced beef, lamb or pork (15% fat)
150ml (5fl oz) red wine
2 x 400g (14oz) cans chopped tomatoes
1 tablespoon tomato purée
salt and pepper

Per serving: 359kcal			
NET CARBS	FIBRE	PROTEIN	FAT
5g	2g	26g	25g

Glossary of UK/US Terms

UK	US
aubergine	eggplant
baking paper	parchment paper
baking/roasting tray	baking/roasting pan
beetroot	beets
bicarbonate of soda	baking soda
biscuit	cookie
celeriac	celery root
chestnut mushrooms	cremini mushrooms
chickpea flour	garbanzo
chickpeas	gram flour
chopping board	cutting board
coriander (fresh)	cilantro
cornflour	cornstarch
courgette	zucchini
dark chocolate	bittersweet chocolate
double cream	heavy cream
flaked almonds	slivered almonds
frying pan	skillet
gherkin	pickle
grill (heat source from above)	broiler
kitchen paper	paper towels
loaf tin	loaf pan
mangetout	snow peas
passata	sieved tomatoes
prawn	shrimp
rapeseed oil	canola oil
red/yellow/green pepper	red/yellow/green bell pepper
rocket	arugula
sieve	strainer
spring onion	scallion
stock	broth
streaky bacon	lean bacon slices
supermarket	grocery store
swede	rutabaga
sweet	candy
take away	takeout
tea towel	dish towel
tin foil	aluminum foil
tomato purée	tomato paste
vegetable mash	mashed vegetables

Index

Social Media

Katie Caldesi is on Instagram and X as @KatieCaldesi and on Facebook under Katie Caldesi's The Good Kitchen Table. Also see her website www.thegoodkitchentable.com. Restaurants and cookery schools can be found at www.caldesi.com or search for Caldesi Italian Restaurants.

Dr David Unwin is on X as @lowcarbGP.

Dr Jen Unwin is on X as @drjenunwin, her website is www.the-chc.org. For further information on carb addiction, see her book *Fork in the Road* (2021).

Jenny Phillips is on Instagram as @jennynutrition and her website is www.inspirednutrition.co.uk.

Resources

The nutritional analysis is only a guide. There are so many variables between nutrition software, ingredients differ around the world and often allowances are not made for fat left at the bottom of a roasting dish, or the size of someone version of a tablespoon! We use www.cronometer.com for the nutritional analysis of the recipes.

Carbs & Cals produces very useful carb and calorie counter books and apps: www.carbsandcals.com.

Freestyle Libre makes instant glucose monitoring systems and can be found at: www.freestylelibre.co.uk.

The Public Health Collaboration is a charity dedicated to informing and implementing healthy decisions for better public health. Find out more at www.phcuk.org.

Diet Doctor has a mass of well researched and evidence-backed information on going low-carb and keto: www.dietdoctor.com.

Research sources from Dr David Unwin's introduction can be found at: www.thegoodkitchentable.com

Acknowledgements

Giancarlo, Jenny and I were delighted to work with Dr David Unwin and Dr Jen Unwin on this project. Their knowledge, experience and help were invaluable. We wish it to be known that they have received no fee for their participation in this book. Instead, we made a donation to the Public Health Collaboration to further their work spreading the real food message.

A massive thank you to publisher Kate Fox; literary agent Jonathan Hayden; editor Scarlet Furness; Maja Smend, for the stunning photography; Lizzie Harris, for the beautiful food styling; Tony Hutchinson for the prop styling; Yasia Williams for the design of the book; and Lisa Pinnell for the production.

Thanks also to Susanne, Bob, Charlotte and Sophie Soin; Debi Peppin and family; Stefano Borella; Gloria Bellugi; Giorgio Caldesi for his fried chicken; Giancarlo and Flavio Caldesi; Louise Ford; and Carly and Robbo Roberts, for your encouragement as well as recipe testing, proofing, shopping, eating and washing up!